Vitamin D - A Novel Therapy for Chronic Diseases?

Edited by

Dimitrios Papandreou

Department of Clinical Nutrition and Dietetics
College of Health Sciences
University of Sharjah
Sharjah
UAE

Vitamin D - A Novel Therapy for Chronic Diseases?

Editor: Dimitrios Papandreou

ISBN (Online): 978-981-5305-33-3

ISBN (Print): 978-981-5305-34-0

ISBN (Paperback): 978-981-5305-35-7

First published in 2024.

need for a court order if at any point you breach any terms of this License Agreement. In no event will any delay or failure by Bentham Science Publishers in enforcing your compliance with this License Agreement constitute a waiver of any of its rights.

3. You acknowledge that you have read this License Agreement, and agree to be bound by its terms and conditions. To the extent that any other terms and conditions presented on any website of Bentham Science Publishers conflict with, or are inconsistent with, the terms and conditions set out in this License Agreement, you acknowledge that the terms and conditions set out in this License Agreement shall prevail.

Bentham Science Publishers Pte. Ltd.
80 Robinson Road #02-00
Singapore 068898
Singapore
Email: subscriptions@benthamscience.net

BENTHAM SCIENCE

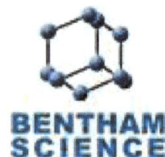

CONTENTS

Shaikha Alnaqbi, Reem El Asmar, Russul AlQutub, Alyaa Masaad, Noor Abu Dheir, Salma Abu Qiyas and *Dimitrios Papandreou*

FOREWORD

In today's swiftly evolving world, where information is abundant and choices are vast, the quest for nutritional wisdom can seem overwhelming. Amid the myriad of dietary trends and the maze of conflicting advice, certain essentials of nutrition emerge as pillars of human health. Prominent among these is vitamin D, a nutrient that has captured the fascination of scientists and the public alike for its critical role in our well-being.

It is my distinct pleasure to present to you a comprehensive exploration of one of the most pivotal vitamins for human health: vitamin D. This book invites you on a journey through the complex world of this remarkable nutrient, shedding light on its crucial functions in the body, its varied sources, and its profound influence on health, with a particular focus on its impact on certain diseases.

The relationship between vitamin D and bone health is widely recognized, yet the scope of its benefits stretches far beyond its role in calcium metabolism. Vitamin D is instrumental in supporting immune function, enhancing mood, and potentially lowering the risk of chronic diseases, captivating researchers, and health professionals with its multifaceted effects. The evolving narrative of vitamin D is one versatility and discovery, with each chapter of research enriching our understanding of its significance.

This book is designed not only as a collection of the latest knowledge but also as a practical guide for those aiming to improve their vitamin D levels. Through clear, evidence-based recommendations and accessible explanations, it equips readers with the tools to make informed health decisions. Whether you are a healthcare professional, a nutrition aficionado, or simply someone interested in the pivotal role of nutrition in health, this book provides valuable insights that can have a lasting impact on your life.

As we venture into the following chapters, let us seize the opportunity to deepen our appreciation for vitamin D, exploring its potential to bolster our health and vitality. May this book illuminate your path to optimal health, serving as a beacon in your pursuit of well-being.

With warm regards

Eleni Andreou, PhD, RDN
Professor of Nutrition
University of Nicosia, Nicosia, Cyprus

PREFACE

The health of the musculoskeletal system depends on vitamin D since it controls the metabolism of calcium and phosphorus. For most people, sunlight with enough ultraviolet B (UVB) radiation is the primary source of it, as it is synthesized in the skin upon exposure. Foods and dietary supplements can also provide it. When exposure to sunlight containing UVB radiation is restricted or limited (as in the winter months), dietary sources become crucial (*e.g.*, due to lack of time spent outdoors or little skin exposure).

Vitamin D is acquired by humans through their food and exposure to sunshine. Vitamin D is found naturally in very few foods. Vitamin D3 is abundant in oily fish, including sardines, salmon, and mackerel. Vitamin D is said to be present in egg yolks, yet the concentrations are somewhat varied. Moreover, egg yolks are a poor source of vitamin D due to their high cholesterol content. Additionally, a few foods—like milk, orange juice, and some bread and cereals—are fortified with vitamin D.

In two hydroxylation steps, vitamin D is transformed into its active metabolite, 1,25-dihydroxyvitamin D (1,25(OH)2D). The primary circulating metabolite of vitamin D, 25(OH)D, is produced in the liver during the first hydroxylation of vitamin D. It is frequently utilized as a biomarker of vitamin D status. In the kidney, 25(OH)D is converted into 1,25(OH)2D during the second hydroxylation. A deficiency of vitamin D is characterized by most specialists as a level of under 20 ng for each milliliter. In 1997, the Institute of Medicine of the US National Academy of Sciences recommended new adequate intakes for vitamin D as 200 IU for children and adults up to 50 years of age, 400 IU for adults 51 to 70 years of age, and 600 IU for adults 71 years of age or older. Vitamin D deficiency can be divided based on UBV, dark skin, being old, and latitude, season, and time of the day of UBV. The other category includes medical/physical conditions or any deficiency, such as fat malabsorption, obesity, chronic kidney disease, and use of medication (*e.g.* anticonvulsant).

The chapters below discuss the most updated research data available on Vitamin D and its relation to several chronic diseases.

Dimitrios Papandreou
Department of Clinical Nutrition and Dietetics
College of Health Sciences
University of Sharjah
Sharjah
UAE

List of Contributors

Alyaa Masaad   Department of Clinical Nutrition and Dietetics, College of Health Sciences, University of Sharjah, Sharjah, UAE

Amina Afrin   Department of Clinical Nutrition and Dietetics, College of Health Sciences, University of Sharjah, Sharjah, UAE

Anam Shakil Kalsekar   Department of Clinical Nutrition and Dietetics, College of Health Sciences, University of Sharjah, Sharjah, UAE

Dimitrios Papandreou   Department of Clinical Nutrition and Dietetics, College of Health Sciences, University of Sharjah, Sharjah, UAE

Khawla Jalal   Department of Clinical Nutrition and Dietetics, College of Health Sciences, University of Sharjah, Sharjah, UAE

May Ali   Department of Clinical Nutrition and Dietetics, College of Health Sciences, University of Sharjah, Sharjah, UAE

Noor Abu Dheir   Department of Clinical Nutrition and Dietetics, College of Health Sciences, University of Sharjah, Sharjah, UAE

Reem El Asmar   Department of Clinical Nutrition and Dietetics, College of Health Sciences, University of Sharjah, Sharjah, UAE

Russul AlQutub   Department of Clinical Nutrition and Dietetics, College of Health Sciences, University of Sharjah, Sharjah, UAE

Rahab Sohail   Department of Clinical Nutrition and Dietetics, College of Health Sciences, University of Sharjah, Sharjah, UAE

Salma Abu Qiyas   Department of Clinical Nutrition and Dietetics, College of Health Sciences, University of Sharjah, Sharjah, UAE

Sheima T. Saleh   Department of Clinical Nutrition and Dietetics, College of Health Sciences, University of Sharjah, Sharjah, UAE

Sharfa Khaleel   Department of Clinical Nutrition and Dietetics, College of Health Sciences, University of Sharjah, Sharjah, UAE

Shaikha Alnaqbi   Department of Clinical Nutrition and Dietetics, College of Health Sciences, University of Sharjah, Sharjah, UAE

CHAPTER 1

History and General Information of Vitamin D

Amina Afrin[1,*], Anam Shakil Kalsekar[1], Khawla Jalal[1], Rahab Sohail[1], Sharfa Khaleel[1], Shaima T. Saleh[1] and Dimitrios Papandreou[1]

[1] *Department of Clinical Nutrition and Dietetics, College of Health Sciences, University of Sharjah, Sharjah, UAE*

Abstract: The historical background of vitamin D for well-being dates to the beginning of the twentieth century. There are two types of vitamin D; ergocalciferol (D2) and cholecalciferol (D3). While D3 is mostly produced in the skin when exposed to sunshine, vitamin D2 is sourced from plant sources and is frequently utilized in fortified meals and supplements. The recommended form of vitamin D for supplementation is D3 since it has a greater potency in elevating and sustaining blood levels of the nutrient. The biochemistry of vitamin D is centered on how it becomes activated in the kidneys and liver to become its active form, which controls the metabolism of phosphorus and calcium. Although ideal serum levels might vary based on personal health considerations, recommended values generally lie between 20 and 50 ng/mL. Egg yolks, fortified dairy products, and fatty fish are good dietary sources of vitamin D; nevertheless, obtaining a sufficient intake only through food may be difficult, necessitating supplementation. However, overindulgence can result in toxicity, which is defined by hypercalcemia and associated symptoms including nausea and weakness. This emphasizes the significance of moderation in supplementing. Because vitamin D is fat-soluble, the body will keep excess rather than quickly excrete it, therefore taking too many supplements can be harmful. While vitamin D is essential for many body processes, getting the right amount of it without running the risk of negative side effects is crucial.

Keywords: Dietary intake, Food sources, Toxicity, Vitamin D history.

INTRODUCTION

Vitamin D is indeed a crucial nutrient for human health, playing a significant role in various physiological processes beyond just bone health. The primary natural source of vitamin D is through the synthesis of cholecalciferol (vitamin D3) in the skin upon exposure to UV-B radiation from sunlight. Vitamin D can also be obtained from dietary sources such as fatty fish (*e.g.*, salmon, mackerel, tuna),

* **Corresponding author Amina Afrin:** Department of Clinical Nutrition and Dietetics, College of Health Sciences, University of Sharjah, Sharjah, UAE; E-mails: U23102372@sharjah.ac.ae, amina.nisthar@gmail.com

fortified foods (*e.g.*, milk, orange juice, cereals), and supplements. Vitamin D plays a crucial role in enhancing the absorption of calcium from the intestines, thereby aiding in maintaining bone health. It regulates calcium and phosphate metabolism, which is essential for bone mineralization and growth. It may also play a role in muscle function and reducing the risk of falls, especially in older adults. Vitamin D also has immunomodulatory effects, influencing both innate and adaptive immune responses. Severe vitamin D deficiency can lead to rickets in children, characterized by skeletal deformities due to impaired mineralization of bones. In adults, severe deficiency can result in osteomalacia, causing weak, soft bones and muscle weakness. Dietary recommendations for vitamin D intake vary by age, sex, and other factors. In the absence of sufficient sunlight exposure, obtaining vitamin D from diet and supplements becomes crucial. While sunlight is a natural source of vitamin D, recommendations regarding sun exposure should balance the benefits of vitamin D synthesis with the risks of skin cancer. Sunscreen use, clothing coverage, time of day, latitude, and skin type all affect the synthesis of vitamin D from sunlight. Overall, maintaining adequate levels of vitamin D is essential for overall health and well-being, and a balanced approach that includes a combination of sunlight exposure, dietary sources, and supplementation when necessary, is recommended.

HISTORY OF VITAMIN D

The story of the discovery of Vitamin D is an interesting one since it was far from a straightforward path. Several lines of research taking place between the 1700s to the 1900s led to its eventual recognition. Since the 1600s, rickets also known as the "English disease", was rampant in different parts of the world, most notably Europe [1, 2]. This time period was marked by the advent of the Industrial revolution bringing in large amounts of air pollution from the burning of fossil fuels and mills, greatly reducing the amount of sunlight available at the ground level. Furthermore, large populations of people migrated into these crowded, air-polluted areas with little to no sunlight exposure. Concurrent to this large-scale migration, was the spread of a new, bone-softening disorder known as 'childhood rickets' when presenting in young children and 'osteomalacia' in adults [3]. Daniel Whistler from the Netherlands was first reported to have described rickets and osteomalacia in 1645 as a condition characterised by a poorly mineralized and deformed skeletal system [1]. Around that time, Franklin Glisson documented lithographic records in his book titled De Rachitide in 1650 featuring children with common symptoms such as bowing of the legs, skeletal deformities, growth retardation, enlargement of the rib cage, head, and muscle weakness [4]. The number of rachitic cases continued to rise till the 1900s. By the 20th century, between 80-90% of the children living in the US and Europe were afflicted with this bone-deforming disorder [5].

A conclusive cure for rickets remained elusive until 19th century when Sniadecki, a Polish physician scientist in 1822 [6], observed that the incidence of rickets differed between children in rural areas exposed to sunlight *versus* those in cities, suggesting that perhaps sunlight might be involved in the etiology of rickets [7]. The 20th century gave rise to much debate surrounding the possible causal factors of rickets which was proposed to be either environmental (in the form of sunlight) or dietary in nature. In 1919, Kurt Huldshinsky [8] made significant contributions to the sunlight-rickets debate by exposing children to UV radiation from a sun quartz lamp. Much to the interest of the scientific community, the X-rays of the children exposed to UV radiation showed marked increases in the mineralization of long bones [9]. It was speculated that the skin exposure to UV rays either from the sun or lamps simulating sunlight, led to a photochemical reaction producing specific products that exerted positive effects on the skeleton. Later many others such as Hess and Weinstock in 1924 experimentally tested the impact of UV irradiation on various inert foods such as lettuce and wheat successfully imparting anti-rachitic properties [10]. In the meantime, some scientists were hypothesizing a dietary etiologic factor for rickets. In 1919, Edward Mellanby, a British biochemist and nutritionist made a landmark observation, that rickets could be induced in dogs by restricting their diet to oatmeal and then reversing the rachitic symptoms by the addition of cod liver oil [11]. This observation indicated that a nutritional deficiency is a probably contributing factor in rickets. The search for the active nutrient responsible for the therapeutic activity of cod liver oil ensued and it was presumed that Vitamin A was responsible.

In Edward Mellanby's words, "Rickets is a deficiency disease which develops in consequence of the absence of some accessory food factor or factors. It, therefore, seems probable that the cause of rickets is a diminished intake of an anti-rachitic factor, which is either [McCollum's] fat-soluble factor A, or has a similar distribution to it" [12]. However, Elmer McCollum refuted that the antirachitic factor was Vitamin A. To test his theory, Elmer and his team conducted an experiment in 1922 wherein cod liver was aerated to oxidise fat-soluble factor A and subsequently heated. Since Vitamin A is highly sensitive to oxidation and heat, it was consequently destroyed in the tested sample of cod liver oil. When fed to rats with xerophthalmia and rickets, findings revealed that cod liver oil maintained its anti-rachitic properties although it lacked Vitamin A's therapeutic impact on xeropthalmia [13]. This phenomenal observation led to the discovery and naming of a new vitamin, Vitamin D. This dichotomy between the separate etiologic factors, namely UV radiation, and diet, served as an impetus to scientifically trace the common denominator. The quandary was settled independently by Harriet Chick [14] and Harry Steenbock [15] at the University of Wisconsin. Steenbock, prompted by this dichotomy, ran a series of experiments, irradiating rats with UV light. He found that the consumption of special foods such as cod liver oil coupled with UV radiation showed an interesting potency to cure rickets [15]. Furthermore, he explained that the anti-rachitic activity was found in the non-saponifiable lipid portion of Vitamin D. The lipid fraction was discovered to be present in diet and skin in the inactive form that can be activated by exposure to UV light [7, 16]. This discovery led to the rapid eradication of rickets as food companies began to fortify foods rich in fats like milk to enhance its anti-rachitic characteristics through irradiation. At this time, however, the chemical makeup of vitamin D was still unknown. Researchers in the 1930s were studying the various members of the cholesterol family in hopes of identifying the chemical structure of Vitamin D [17]. Eventually, Adolf Windaus who was working extensively in clarifying the structures of various sterols, elucidated that 7-dehydrocholestrol is the precursor of vitamin D in the skin [18]. Windaus named the newly found form of vitamin D vitamin D3. In 1928, he received the Nobel Prize for his work on sterols and the vitamins associated with them. By 1930s, chemically synthesized forms of vitamin D, such as vitamin D3 was available. This opened the door for research to shed light on the various active forms of vitamin D, its metabolism, biological roles, serum levels, recommended amounts for optimal health and sources of vitamin D.

Types of Vitamin D

Vitamin D, or calciferol, constitutes a group of fat-soluble seco-sterols. Vitamin D analogs encompass both natural and synthetic forms of the vitamin, each with distinct chemical compositions and origins, with the two primary variants being vitamin D2 (ergocalciferol) and vitamin D3 (cholecalciferol) [19]. The natural analogs, or vitamins, include Vitamin D1, D2, D3, D4, and D5. Vitamin D1 is a molecular compound of ergocalciferol (D2) and lumisterol in a 1:1 ratio [20].

Vitamin D2 primarily derives from plant-based sources such as mushrooms and fortified foods. It is largely synthesized commercially by irradiating ergosterol, a sterol in certain fungi and yeast, with ultraviolet light. Following ingestion, vitamin D2 undergoes hydroxylation processes in the liver and kidneys to produce calcitriol, the biologically active form of vitamin D2, albeit with lower efficiency than the other common form of vitamin D, vitamin D3 [21].

Contrary to vitamin D2, vitamin D3 is predominantly sourced from animal products and synthesized endogenously in the skin upon exposure to ultraviolet B radiation. The synthesis begins with converting 7-dehydrocholesterol in the skin to pre-vitamin D3, subsequently transforming into vitamin D3. This endogenous production mechanism is highly efficient and serves as the primary source of vitamin D3 for human populations [22].

Both vitamin D3 and D2 are commercially synthesized and can be found in supplements or fortified foods. Despite differences in their side chain structures, the metabolic pathways of D2 and D3 remain unaffected, with both forms serving as prohormones upon activation [19]. Moreover, both variants exhibit efficient absorption within the small intestine, achieved through straightforward passive diffusion and a mechanism mediated by carrier proteins in the intestinal membrane [23].

A recent systematic review of randomized and non-randomized controlled studies involving a total of 1,277 healthy human participants from 24 studies investigated the comparative effectiveness of vitamin D2 and D3 in increasing the concentrations of vitamin D metabolites in the bloodstream and influencing various functional indicators, such as serum parathyroid hormone (PTH) levels, isometric muscle strength, hand grip strength, and bone mineral density. The results indicated a notable difference in efficacy between cholecalciferol and ergocalciferol. Cholecalciferol demonstrated higher effectiveness in improving total 25-hydroxyvitamin D (25(OH)D) levels and reducing PTH levels compared to ergocalciferol. Further analysis through meta-regression revealed that the difference in efficacy between cholecalciferol and ergocalciferol was less pronounced at lower doses. Interestingly, the average daily dose emerged as a significant predictor of effect size, suggesting that dosage plays a crucial role in determining the magnitude of the intervention's impact [24].

In addition to vitamin D2 and D3, there are less studied forms, such as vitamin D4 (22-dihydroergocalciferol) and vitamin D5 (sitocalciferol). Vitamin D4 is structurally similar to D2 and D3 and is found in fish liver oils and certain mushrooms. However, its physiological significance is less researched. Similarly, vitamin D5 is found in specific plant sources, but its biological activity and metabolism are poorly understood compared to D2 and D3. Alongside natural forms, synthetic analogs of vitamin D, including Maxacalcitol, Calcipotriol, Dihydrotachysterol (DHT), Paricalcitol, Tacalcitol, Doxercalciferol, and Falecalcitriol, offer various therapeutic potentials and applications, expanding the utilization of vitamin D in healthcare [20].

Biology of Vitamin D

Vitamin D is comprised of an active form, calcitriol, which binds to the vitamin D receptor (VDR), which is a specialized protein that is commonly found in some specific cells within their nuclei. The VDR operates as a transcription factor due to the binding interaction, which prompts the expression of numerous genes that play a key role in crucial processes such as calcium absorption, which occurs in the intestines [25]. The VDR is expressed in a range of organs across the body, considering the fact that it is a member of the nuclear receptor superfamily, which is indicative of the active role that vitamin D plays in physiological functions [26]. In order for the body to maintain and optimize calcium and phosphorus levels within the bloodstream, VDR is usually activated in crucial cells in the bones, parathyroid gland, and intestines, together with other crucial hormones such as calcitonin and parathyroid hormone.

Bone density and integrity regulation in addition to overall skeletal health, are optimized through VDR activation, even though its impact also facilitates crucial functions in immune functioning and cellular proliferation. The impact of vitamin D on bone health and well-being is associated with the occurrence of conditions like rickets in situations where there is a deficiency of the vital nutrients, especially during the formative years of early childhood. The role of vitamin D in immune regulation is evident considering the fact that monocytes and T lymphocytes in addition to some other white blood cells, express VDR [25]. Bone metabolism is also a crucial process that is attributable to VDR, even though the vitamin also impacts crucial physiological processes such as tyrosine hydroxylase gene expression within adrenal medullary cells [27]. Vitamin D also facilitates the synthesis of neurotrophic factors and hence highlighting the extensive role it plays in both homeostasis and cellular function.

The influence of vitamin D on vascular function and its regularization of blood pressure enhances cardiovascular health [26]. The biological activation of vitamin D is initiated by hydroxylation in the liver to convert it to 25-hydroxyvitamin D, and a second hydroxylation occurs in the kidneys to further convert it into its active form, which is crucial for exerting the effects of vitamin D receptors after binding with them [28]. The stimulation of calcium-binding proteins to facilitate the transportation of the vital mineral into the bloodstream from intestinal epithelial cells is enhanced by vitamin D, which is crucial for facilitating calcium homeostasis [29]. VDR is also vital for enhancing cell growth and differentiation in the body by regulating gene expression that is vital for cell cycle control and cellular differentiation, which may lead to benefits such as the exertion of anti-cancer effects.

While the parathyroid hormone and blood phosphate levels play a key role in regulating the conversion of vitamin D to its active form, the synthesis of the vital nutrient is regulated by numerous factors which include latitude, skin pigmentation, and seasons. Vitamin D status is best assessed by the evaluation of serum levels with sufficient levels typically being above 30ng/mL, while inadequate levels being anything that is below 20ng/mL [30].

Recommendations on Serum Levels of Vitamin D

Depending on factors like age, sex and others, different authorities have different recommendations for appropriate serum levels of 25(OH)D [48]. Many vitamin D specialists believe that blood 25(OH)D concentrations above 100 nmol/L are ideal for all health outcomes, including bone [31]. According to an analysis published in 2014, blood levels of 25(OH)D that were most beneficial for all outcomes seemed to be around 30 ng/mL (75 nmol/L) [32]. For age group 1- 70 years, World Health Organization (WHO) recommends an intake of 200 IU/d, and European Food Safety Authority (EFA) recommends 600 IU/d [33]. According to the Endocrine Society, adults may require around 1,500–2,000 IU of vitamin D per day, while children and adolescents may require at least 1,000 IU per day in order to maintain blood 25(OH)D levels above 75 nmol/L (30 ng/mL) [34]. On the other hand, the government of the United Kingdom advises its residents who are four years of age and older to consume 10 mcg (400 IU) daily [47]. The Endocrine Society deemed a level of up to 250 nmol/L to be safe and suggested a preferable range of 100–150 nmol/L for 25(OH)D [34]. Additionally, the Endocrine Society determined that vitamin D intoxication is a very uncommon condition that is typically not noticed until blood levels of 25(OH)D exceed 375 nmol/L [35].

During pregnancy, IOM (a), EFSA (b), SACN (c), and WHO (d) recommended an intake of 600 IU/d (a &b), 400 IU/d (c), and 200 IU/d (d) of vitamin D, respectively [33, 47]. Hollis and Wagner reported that pregnant women who consumed 4000 IU/d during pregnancy were able to sustain circulating levels of 25(OH)D in the range of 100–125 nmol/L without having any adverse effects [36]. According to certain observational studies, maternal serum 25(OH)D concentrations below 75 nmol/L have been repeatedly linked to an increased risk of pregnancy problems, such as preterm birth, preeclampsia, gestational diabetes, small for gestational age newborns, and bacterial vaginosis [37]. Preterm birth rates can be lowered by over half with an intake of 4000 IU/d during pregnancy, according to Wagner *et al.* [38]. This same level of intake may also lessen other pregnancy-related complications like preeclampsia, gestational diabetes, and potentially postpartum haemorrhage [39, 40].

The recommended serum level of 25(OH)D for athletes is > 32 ng/mL while the preferred one is > 40 ng/mL [41]. According to numerous studies, a significant percentage of athletes have vitamin D insufficiency or deficiency in the measured levels of vitamin D in different types of sports [42]. Hypovitaminosis D was found to be frequent among National Basketball Association players. It has been reported that professional baskletball players had deficiency (<20 ng/mL) and insufficiency (20–30 ng/mL) at 32.3% and 41.2%, respectively [43]. Athletes may have low vitamin D levels due to a variety of factors, such as racing, decreased synthesis of vitamin D by the skin from sunlight, and inadequate dietary vitamin D intake [44].

With regard to infants, as recommended by the IOM and later confirmed by the AAP the appropriate serum level is at least 20 ng/mL for both preterm and full-term respectivelly [45]. For most full-term newborns, dosages of 400 IU/day of vitamin D3 were adequate to reach 25(OH)D concentrations > 50 nmol/L [46]. Moreover, the Endocrine Society recommends supplementing infants up to one year old with 400–1000 IU/d [31].

The best method to determine the ideal dosage is to customize it for each individual by taking a serum 25(OH)D measurement and modifying the vitamin D dosage to reach 25(OH)D levels between 75 and 250 nmol/L [31]. There are various strategies to maintain vitamin D sufficiency and to treat deficiency. For eight weeks, the Endocrine Society advises taking 50,000 IU of vitamin D every week followed by an intake of 50,000 IU every two weeks in order to maintain vitamin D sufficiency. To achieve a new steady-state level of 25(OH)D, it typically takes 8–12 weeks for people who choose to take vitamin D daily. It has been reported that circulating levels of 25(OH)D would rise with every 100 IU/d consumed and will stabilise at 1.5–2.5 nmol/L after 8–12 weeks. As a result, healthy people of normal weight who consume 2000 IU/d are expected to maintain circulating levels of 25(OH)D between 75 and 100 nmol/L. Individuals who consume 5000 IU/d will be able to raise and maintain blood levels between 100 and 150 nmol/L [31].

Dietary Intake

The National Academy of Medicine published dietary reference intakes for vitamin D that replaced earlier guidelines that were stated based on adequate intake. The guidelines were developed with the assumption that the person's lack of skin synthesis of vitamin D is the result of insufficient sun exposure. The recommended intake for vitamin D is the total amount obtained from food, drink, and supplements, and it is based on the assumption that calcium needs are being satisfied as presented in the Table **1** below [49].

Food Sources

Few foods naturally contain vitamin D, although it is frequently added as a fortifier in manufactured food items. Certain nations artificially add vitamin D fortification to their primary foods.

Table 1. Recommended intake for vitamin D.

Age group	RDA (IU/day)	(µg/day)
Infants 0–12 months	400	10
1–70 years	600	15
Adults > 70 years	800	20
Pregnant/Lactating	600	15

Institute for Medicine, 2011 [49].

Natural Sources

Generally speaking, foods derived from animals—fish, meat, offal, eggs, and dairy—contain vitamin D3 [50]. Fungal ergosterol is exposed to UV light to create vitamin D2 [51]. When exposed to UV light, mushrooms and the lichen Cladina arbuscula grow in vitamin D2 [52]. Industrial ultraviolet lamps are one way to encourage this process for fortification. Vitamin D2 and D3 are reported are reported by the US Department of Agriculture as a single number.

Food Fortification and Preparation

Some examples of fortified foods with vitamin D include fruit juices, energy bars, soy protein-based beverages, specific cheeses and cheese products as well as flour products [53, 54]. Cooking such as boiling, frying and baking may enhance loss of Vitamin D up to 30% cont [55].

Toxicity/Excess of Vitamin D

There has been a significant increase in the trend of prescribing vitamin D, which might cause hypervitaminosis D. It is often underestimated, despite its significance [56]. Hypervitaminosis D is an uncommon condition, and it rarely arises from foods that are rich in vitamin D, such as fish, meat, and dairy products. Additionally, excessive sun exposure does not lead to high levels of vitamin D due to its regulation and conversion into inactive metabolites. Vitamin D toxicity typically arises from exceeding the recommended amount of vitamin D in fortified foods or supplements. This is often due to the improper use of over-the-counter supplements, incorrect prescriptions, or inadequate supervision in individuals who need high dosages for the treatment of conditions such as osteoporosis, surgery, renal osteodystrophy, gastric bypass, psoriasis, celiac disease, or inflammatory bowel disease. The condition of hypervitaminosis could cause hypercalcemia and disrupt the regulation of bone metabolism [57].

According to Jones and his colleagues, there are three primary theories that explain the mechanisms behind vitamin D toxicity. All of these ideas are based on the theory that high levels of vitamin D metabolites in the bloodstream cause nuclear VDR to become active in some cells, which then sets off the transcriptional machinery [58].

As per the 2011 National Academy of Medicine Report, acute vitamin D toxicity often occurs when vitamin D doses exceed 10,000 IU/day, leading to blood 25(OH)D concentrations above 150 ng/mL. while chronic vitamin D toxicity occurs with prolonged use of dosages over 4000 IU/day, resulting in 25(OH)D values ranging from 50 to 150 ng/mL [59]. Up to 4000 IU/day (or equal monthly) is safe for most people, according to most research [60]. A retrospective analysis of U.S. National Poison Data System data shows a significant increase in toxic vitamin D exposure from 196 cases per year from 2000–2005 to 4535 exposures per year from 2005–2011, despite significantly higher total exposures [61]. No deaths occurred, with 2 to 22 patients each year experiencing adverse medical consequences (major or moderate). The number of exposures increased significantly, but serious effects were rare [62]. In addition, a study conducted in Minnesota found that the occurrence of 25(OH)D levels above 50 ng/mL increased from 9 to 233 cases per 100,000 person-years between 2002 and 2011, and there was no clear evidence of a corresponding rise in acute clinical toxicity [63]. A separate investigation conducted in the United States revealed that out of a total of 60,237 25(OH)D tests, only 27 had 25(OH)D concentrations exceeding 150 ng/mL [64]. In contrast, a study conducted in Pakistan with a sample size of 2249 children revealed that 64% of the children had serum 25(OH)D concentrations below 30 ng/mL. However, it was observed that 9.8% and 3.2% of the children had concentrations above 80 and 150 ng/mL, respectively. These percentages were significantly higher than those reported in studies conducted in the United States [65].

In an RCT, 163 Caucasian women aged 57-90 with a baseline 25(OH)D level below 20 ng/mL were given oral vitamin D ranging from 400 to 4800 IU/day and calcium citrate as a dietary supplement to achieve a daily intake of 1200 mg. At three months, 8.8% of individuals experienced hypercalcemia (more than 10.2 mg/dL), and 30.6% had hypercalciuria (exceeding 300 mg/day). Hypercalciuria was temporary in 50% of the participants, persistent in the remaining half, and prevalent in the placebo group, making it uncertain whether calcium, vitamin D, or both were responsible for it [66]. Another RCT, conducted in Canada, investigated the effect of vitamin D dosages on volumetric bone mineral density and strength in 311 healthy individuals aged 55-70. The participants had initial 25-hydroxyvitamin D levels ranging from 12 to 50 ng/mL, with an average of 31 ng/mL. Vitamin D3 dosages of 400, 4,000, or 10,000 IU daily were administered to participants at random for three years. The diet was enriched with 1200 mg/day of calcium. 25(OH)D levels increased in a manner that was dependent on the dosage. Administering Vitamin D3 at doses of 4000 or 10,000 IU/day for 3 years resulted in a statistically significant reduction in radial volumetric BMD but did not impact bone strength in the radius or tibia. The study concluded that there is no support for recommending high-dose vitamin D supplementation (≥4000 IU/day) for bone health, and any negative effects need further investigation [67]. Supplementation is a primary factor that might lead to potentially harmful levels of 25(OH)D. The condition can be prevented with cautious use of vitamin D supplements and persistent monitoring [56].

CONCLUSION

To conclude, biological processes in the human body highlight the importance of vitamin D for multifaceted roles. Serum recommendations provide benchmarks for good health, but achieving optimum levels continues to be challenging. Even though vitamin D may be found in certain natural food sources, it is sometimes required to be taken as a dietary supplementary form to reach the suggested levels. Vitamin D overdose can have negative consequences, so care must be taken to prevent toxicity. Even though this vital vitamin has many health benefits, moderation is crucial to get all these benefits without suffering from side effects.

REFERENCES

[1]   Whistler D. De morbo puerili anglorum, quem patrio idiômate indigenae vocant The rickets: Ex officina Wilhemi Christiani Boxii.

[2]   Bouillon R, Antonio L. Nutritional rickets: Historic overview and plan for worldwide eradication. J Steroid Biochem Mol Biol 2020; 198: 105563.
[http://dx.doi.org/10.1016/j.jsbmb.2019.105563] [PMID: 31809867]

[3]   Rajakumar K, Greenspan SL, Thomas SB. Holick MFJAjoph. SOLAR ultraviolet radiation and vitamin D: a historical perspective. 2007; 97(10): 1746-54.

[4]   Glisson FJTrdt. De rachitide, sive morbo puerili, qui vulgo. 1650.

[5]   Holick MFJTJoci. Resurrection of vitamin D deficiency and rickets. 2006; 116(8): 2062-72.

[6]   Sniadecki SJJ, Sniadecki JJN. on the cure of rickets.(1840) Cited by W. Mozolowski 1939; 143: 121-4.

[7]   Jones G. The discovery and synthesis of the nutritional factor vitamin D. Int J Paleopathol 2018; 23: 96-9.
[http://dx.doi.org/10.1016/j.ijpp.2018.01.002] [PMID: 30573171]

[8]   Huldschinsky K. Heilung von Rachitis durch künstliche Höhensonne. Dtsch Med Wochenschr 1919; 45(26): 712-3.
[http://dx.doi.org/10.1055/s-0028-1137830]

[9]   Huldschinsky C. The ultra-violet light treatment of rickets: Sollux publishing company; 1926.

[10]   Hess AF, Weinstock MJJoBC. Antirachitic properties imparted to inert fluids and to green vegetables by ultra-violet irradiation. 1924; 62(2): 301-13.

[11] Mellanby EJNr. An experimental investigation on rickets. 1976; 34(11): 338-40.

[12] Mellanby EJBmj. A British Medical Association lecture on deficiency diseases, with special reference to rickets. 1924; 1(3308): 895.

[13] McCollum EV, Simmonds N, Becker JE, Shipley PJJoBC. Studies on experimental rickets: XXI. An experimental demonstration of the existence of a vitamin which promotes calcium deposition. 1922; 53(2): 293-312.

[14] Chick H, Roscoe MHJBJ. Influence of diet and sunlight upon the amount of vitamin A and vitamin D in the milk afforded by a cow. 1926; 20(3): 632.

[15] Steenbock H, Black AJJoBC. Fat-soluble vitamins: XVII. The induction of growth-promoting and calcifying properties in a ration by exposure to ultra-violet light. 1924; 61(2): 405-22.

[16] Gallagher JC, Rosen CJJTLD, Endocrinology. Vitamin D: 100 years of discoveries, yet controversy continues. 2023; 11(5): 362-74.

[17] Wolf G. The discovery of vitamin D: the contribution of Adolf Windaus. J Nutr 2004; 134(6): 1299-302.
[http://dx.doi.org/10.1093/jn/134.6.1299] [PMID: 15173387]

[18] Windaus A, Linsert O, Luttringhaus WGJAdC. Ulberdas kristalline Vitamin D 2. 1932; 492: 226-41.

[19] Del Valle HB, Yaktine AL, Taylor CL, Ross AC. Dietary reference intakes for calcium and vitamin D. 2011.

[20] Nair R, Maseeh A, Vitamin D. Vitamin D: The "sunshine" vitamin. J Pharmacol Pharmacother 2012; 3(2): 118-26.
[PMID: 22629085]

[21] Bikle DD. Vitamin D metabolism, mechanism of action, and clinical applications. Chem Biol 2014; 21(3): 319-29.
[http://dx.doi.org/10.1016/j.chembiol.2013.12.016] [PMID: 24529992]

[22] Wilson LR, Tripkovic L, Hart KH, Lanham-New SA. Vitamin D deficiency as a public health issue: using vitamin D $_2$ or vitamin D $_3$ in future fortification strategies. Proc Nutr Soc 2017; 76(3): 392-9.
[http://dx.doi.org/10.1017/S0029665117000349] [PMID: 28347378]

[23] Silva MC, Furlanetto TW. Intestinal absorption of vitamin D: a systematic review. Nutr Rev 2018; 76(1): 60-76.
[http://dx.doi.org/10.1093/nutrit/nux034] [PMID: 29025082]

[24] Balachandar R, Pullakhandam R, Kulkarni B, Sachdev HS. Relative Efficacy of Vitamin D$_2$ and Vitamin D$_3$ in Improving Vitamin D Status: Systematic Review and Meta-Analysis. Nutrients 2021; 13(10): 3328.
[http://dx.doi.org/10.3390/nu13103328] [PMID: 34684328]

[25] Voltan G, Cannito M, Ferrarese M, Ceccato F, Camozzi V. Vitamin D: An overview of gene regulation, ranging from metabolism to genomic effects. Genes (Basel) 2023; 14(9): 1691-1.
[http://dx.doi.org/10.3390/genes14091691] [PMID: 37761831]

[26] Bastyte D, Tamasauskiene L, Golubickaite I, Ugenskiene R, Sitkauskiene B. Vitamin D receptor and vitamin D binding protein gene polymorphisms in patients with asthma: a pilot study. BMC Pulm Med 2023; 23(1): 245.
[http://dx.doi.org/10.1186/s12890-023-02531-3]

[27] Usategui-Martín R, De Luis-Román DA, Fernández-Gómez JM, Ruiz-Mambrilla M, Pérez-Castrillón JL, Vitamin D. Vitamin D receptor (*VDR*) gene polymorphisms modify the response to vitamin D supplementation: A systematic review and meta-analysis. Nutrients 2022; 14(2): 360.
[http://dx.doi.org/10.3390/nu14020360] [PMID: 35057541]

[28] Hussain S, Yates C, Campbell MJ. Vitamin D and Systems Biology. Nutrients 2022; 14(24): 5197.

[http://dx.doi.org/10.3390/nu14245197] [PMID: 36558356]

[29]   Falzone L. Role of vitamin D in health and disease: how diet may improve vitamin D absorption. Int J Food Sci Nutr 2023; 74(2): 121-3.
[http://dx.doi.org/10.1080/09637486.2023.2199179] [PMID: 37057375]

[30]   Haq A, Ahsan N. Vitamin D Deficiency, Biology and its Functions. 2020. Available from: https://www.actascientific.com/ASNH/pdf/ASNH-04-0783.pdf

[31]   Kimball SM, Holick MF. Official recommendations for vitamin D through the life stages in developed countries. Eur J Clin Nutr 2020; 74(11): 1514-8.
[http://dx.doi.org/10.1038/s41430-020-00706-3] [PMID: 32820241]

[32]   Bischoff-Ferrari HA. Optimal Serum 25-Hydroxyvitamin D Levels for Multiple Health Outcomes. Sunlight, Vitamin D and Skin Cancer. 55-71.

[33]   Dietary reference values for vitamin D. EFSA J 2016; 14(10): e04547.
[http://dx.doi.org/10.2903/j.efsa.2016.4547]

[34]   Holick MF, Binkley NC, Bischoff-Ferrari HA, *et al.* Evaluation, treatment, and prevention of vitamin D deficiency: an Endocrine Society clinical practice guideline. J Clin Endocrinol Metab 2011; 96(7): 1911-30.
[http://dx.doi.org/10.1210/jc.2011-0385] [PMID: 21646368]

[35]   Manson JE, Cook NR, Lee IM, *et al.* Vitamin D supplements and prevention of cancer and cardiovascular disease. N Engl J Med 2019; 380(1): 33-44.
[http://dx.doi.org/10.1056/NEJMoa1809944] [PMID: 30415629]

[36]   Hollis BW, Johnson D, Hulsey TC, Ebeling M, Wagner CL. Vitamin D supplementation during pregnancy: Double-blind, randomized clinical trial of safety and effectiveness. J Bone Miner Res 2011; 26(10): 2341-57.
[http://dx.doi.org/10.1002/jbmr.463] [PMID: 21706518]

[37]   Karras SN, Wagner CL, Castracane VD. Understanding vitamin D metabolism in pregnancy: From physiology to pathophysiology and clinical outcomes. Metabolism 2018; 86: 112-23.
[http://dx.doi.org/10.1016/j.metabol.2017.10.001] [PMID: 29066285]

[38]   Wagner CL, Baggerly C, McDonnell S, *et al.* Post-hoc analysis of vitamin D status and reduced risk of preterm birth in two vitamin D pregnancy cohorts compared with South Carolina March of Dimes 2009–2011 rates. J Steroid Biochem Mol Biol 2016; 155(Pt B): 245-51.
[http://dx.doi.org/10.1016/j.jsbmb.2015.10.022] [PMID: 26554936]

[39]   Rodrigues MRK, Lima SAM, Mazeto GMFS, *et al.* Efficacy of vitamin D supplementation in gestational diabetes mellitus: Systematic review and meta-analysis of randomized trials. PLoS One 2019; 14(3): e0213006.
[http://dx.doi.org/10.1371/journal.pone.0213006] [PMID: 30901325]

[40]   Palacios C, Kostiuk LK, Peña-Rosas JP. Vitamin D supplementation for women during pregnancy. Cochrane Libr 2019; 2019(7).
[http://dx.doi.org/10.1002/14651858.CD008873.pub4]

[41]   Yoon S, Kwon O, Kim J. Vitamin D in athletes: focus on physical performance and musculoskeletal injuries. Phys Act Nutr 2021; 25(2): 20-5.
[http://dx.doi.org/10.20463/pan.2021.0011] [PMID: 34315203]

[42]   Bezuglov E, Tikhonova A, Zueva A, *et al.* Prevalence and treatment of vitamin D deficiency in young male russian soccer players in winter. Nutrients 2019; 11(10): 2405.
[http://dx.doi.org/10.3390/nu11102405] [PMID: 31597404]

[43]   Grieshober JA, Mehran N, Photopolous C, *et al.* Vitamin D insufficiency among professional basketball players: A relationship to fracture risk and athletic performance. Orthop J Sports Med 2018; 6(5).
[http://dx.doi.org/10.1177/2325967118774329] [PMID: 29845086]

[44]   Williams K, Askew C, Mazoue C, Guy J, Torres-McGehee TM, Jackson JB III. Vitamin D3 supplementation and stress fractures in high-risk collegiate athletes – a pilot study. Orthop Res Rev 2020; 12: 9-17.
[http://dx.doi.org/10.2147/ORR.S233387] [PMID: 32161507]

[45]   Roth DE, Abrams SA, Aloia J, *et al.* Global prevalence and disease burden of vitamin D deficiency: a roadmap for action in low- and middle-income countries. Ann N Y Acad Sci 2018; 1430(1): 44-79.
[http://dx.doi.org/10.1111/nyas.13968] [PMID: 30225965]

[46]   Zittermann A, Pilz S, Berthold HK. Serum 25-hydroxyvitamin D response to vitamin D supplementation in infants: a systematic review and meta-analysis of clinical intervention trials. Eur J Nutr 2020; 59(1): 359-69.
[http://dx.doi.org/10.1007/s00394-019-01912-x] [PMID: 30721411]

[47]   Available from: https://www.bing.com/search?q= Scientific+Advisory+Committee+on+Nutrition.+ Vitamin+D+and+Healthexternal+link+disclaimer.+2016.&cvid=972fb439bdbf4f63b0c84545e568b28 0&gs_lcrp=EgZjaHJvbWUyBggAEEUYODIBBzgyM2owajSoAgCwAgA&FORM=ANAB01&PC=A CTS

[48]   Available from: https://ods.od.nih.gov/factsheets/VitaminD-HealthProfessional/

[49]   IOM (Institute of Medicine). Dietary Reference Intakes for Calcium and Vitamin D. A Catharine Ross, Christine L Taylor, Ann L Yaktine and HBDV, editor. Washington, DC: The National Academies Press; 2011.

[50]   Schmid A, Walther B. Natural vitamin D content in animal products. Adv Nutr 2013; 4(4): 453-62.
[http://dx.doi.org/10.3945/an.113.003780] [PMID: 23858093]

[51]   Keegan RJH, Lu Z, Bogusz JM, Williams JE, Holick MF. Photobiology of vitamin D in mushrooms and its bioavailability in humans. Dermatoendocrinol 2013; 5(1): 165-76.
[http://dx.doi.org/10.4161/derm.23321] [PMID: 24494050]

[52]   Wang T, Bengtsson G, Kärnefelt I, Björn LO. Provitamins and vitamins D2 and D3 in Cladina spp. over a latitudinal gradient: possible correlation with UV levels. J Photochem Photobiol B 2001; 62(1-2): 118-22.
[http://dx.doi.org/10.1016/S1011-1344(01)00160-9] [PMID: 11693362]

[53]   De Lourdes Samaniego-Vaesken M, Alonso-Aperte E, Varela-Moreiras G. Vitamin food fortification today. Food Nutr Res 2012; 56(1): 5459.
[http://dx.doi.org/10.3402/fnr.v56i0.5459] [PMID: 22481896]

[54]   Spiro A, Buttriss JL, Vitamin D. Vitamin D : An overview of vitamin D status and intake in E urope. Nutr Bull 2014; 39(4): 322-50.
[http://dx.doi.org/10.1111/nbu.12108] [PMID: 25635171]

[55]   Jakobsen J, Knuthsen P. Stability of vitamin D in foodstuffs during cooking. Food Chem 2014; 148: 170-5.
[http://dx.doi.org/10.1016/j.foodchem.2013.10.043] [PMID: 24262542]

[56]   Muneer S, Siddiqui I, Majid H, Zehra N, Jafri L, Khan AH. Practices of vitamin D supplementation leading to vitamin D toxicity: Experience from a Low-Middle Income Country. Ann Med Surg (Lond) 2022; 73(Jan): 103227.
[http://dx.doi.org/10.1016/j.amsu.2021.103227] [PMID: 35079366]

[57]   Asif A, Farooq N. Vitamin D Toxicity. 2024.

[58]   Janoušek J, Pilařová V, Macáková K, *et al.* Vitamin D: sources, physiological role, biokinetics, deficiency, therapeutic use, toxicity, and overview of analytical methods for detection of vitamin D and its metabolites. Crit Rev Clin Lab Sci 2022; 59(8): 517-54.
[http://dx.doi.org/10.1080/10408363.2022.2070595] [PMID: 35575431]

[59]   Dominguez LJ, Farruggia M, Veronese N, Barbagallo M, Vitamin D. Vitamin D Sources, Metabolism,

and Deficiency: Available Compounds and Guidelines for Its Treatment. Metabolites 2021; 11(4): 255.
[http://dx.doi.org/10.3390/metabol1040255] [PMID: 33924215]

[60]　Rosen CJ, Gallagher JC. The 2011 IOM report on vitamin D and calcium requirements for north america: clinical implications for providers treating patients with low bone mineral density. Journal of clinical densitometry: The official journal of the International Society for Clinical Densitometry. 2011; 14(2): 79–84.

[61]　Khaw KT, Stewart AW, Waayer D, *et al.* Effect of monthly high-dose vitamin D supplementation on falls and non-vertebral fractures: secondary and post-hoc outcomes from the randomised, double-blind, placebo-controlled ViDA trial. Lancet Diabetes Endocrinol 2017; 5(6): 438-47.
[http://dx.doi.org/10.1016/S2213-8587(17)30103-1] [PMID: 28461159]

[62]　Spiller HA, Good TF, Spiller NE, Aleguas A. Vitamin D exposures reported to US poison centers 2000–2014. Hum Exp Toxicol 2016; 35(5): 457-61.
[http://dx.doi.org/10.1177/0960327115595685] [PMID: 26519481]

[63]　Dudenkov D v, Yawn BP, Oberhelman SS, *et al.* Changing Incidence of Serum 25-Hydroxyvitamin D Values Above 50 ng/mL: A 10-Year Population-Based Study. Mayo Clinic proceedings. 2015; 90(5): 577–86.

[64]　Genzen JR, Gosselin JT, Wilson TC, Racila E, Krasowski MD. Analysis of vitamin D status at two academic medical centers and a national reference laboratory: result patterns vary by age, gender, season, and patient location. BMC Endocr Disord 2013; 13(1): 52.
[http://dx.doi.org/10.1186/1472-6823-13-52] [PMID: 24188187]

[65]　Khan AH, Majid H, Iqbal R. Shifting of vitamin D deficiency to hypervitaminosis and toxicity. J Coll Physicians Surg Pak 2014; 24(7): 536.
[PMID: 25052986]

[66]　Gallagher JC, Smith LM, Yalamanchili V. Incidence of hypercalciuria and hypercalcemia during vitamin D and calcium supplementation in older women. Menopause 2014; 21(11): 1173-80.
[http://dx.doi.org/10.1097/GME.0000000000000270] [PMID: 24937025]

[67]　Burt LA, Billington EO, Rose MS, Raymond DA, Hanley DA, Boyd SK. Effect of high-dose vitamin d supplementation on volumetric bone density and bone strength. JAMA 2019; 322(8): 736-45.
[http://dx.doi.org/10.1001/jama.2019.11889] [PMID: 31454046]

CHAPTER 2

Vitamin D, Immunity, and Gut Health

Russul AlQutub[1,*], **Reem El Asmar**[1] and **Dimitrios Papandreou**[1]

[1] *Department of Clinical Nutrition and Dietetics, College of Health Sciences, University of Sharjah, Sharjah, UAE*

Abstract: The gut microbiota, a complex bacterial community within the gastrointestinal system, critically regulates human physiology. This article explores the complex interactions between the gut microbiota and vitamin D, impacting immunity and overall health. Vitamin D plays a role in immunological modulation, cell proliferation, and maintaining intestinal balance highlighting the intricate connections between gut microbiota and vitamin D in the gastrointestinal system. Recent research indicates that vitamin D receptors in the gastrointestinal tract may influence the gut microbiota's composition. Dysbiosis, an imbalance in the gut microbiota, is linked to various illnesses, including autoimmune diseases and metabolic disorders. This section examines the effects of low vitamin D levels on immunity, associating insufficient amounts with increased susceptibility to infections and autoimmune diseases like rheumatoid arthritis, multiple sclerosis, and Hashimoto's thyroiditis. Conversely, studies demonstrate that immune function relies on maintaining adequate vitamin D levels, particularly through calcitriol, the active form of vitamin D, regulating innate and adaptive immunity. Epidemiological research supports the hypothesis that sufficient vitamin D levels could reduce the prevalence of illnesses, including autoimmune diseases and osteoporosis. The chapter underscores the potential preventive benefits of adequate vitamin D intake, reviewing data from research on multiple sclerosis, Hashimoto's illness, and rheumatoid arthritis.

In conclusion, this exploration highlights vitamin D's critical role in immune system performance, gut health, and microbiota composition. While existing studies suggest the potential benefits of vitamin D for autoimmune illnesses, further research is imperative to establish conclusive evidence, especially regarding vitamin D supplementation for these ailments.

Keywords: Autoimmune disorders, Gut microbiota, Immunity, Microbiome-health relationship, Vitamin D.

* **Corresponding author Russul AlQutub:** Department of Clinical Nutrition and Dietetics, College of Health Sciences, University of Sharjah, Sharjah, UAE; E-mails: U23102372@sharjah.ac.ae, rbq97@yahoo.com

INTRODUCTION

The gut microbiota, composed of microorganisms including bacteria, viruses, and fungi, resides within the gastrointestinal (GI) tract [1]. Nowadays, there is a growing recognition of the microbiota's significance in human physiology, leading some to regard it as a distinct organ within the body [2]. Moreover, emerging evidence highlights its pivotal role in influencing human health and the development of diseases. The gut microbiota serves crucial functions in maintaining metabolic and immune well-being, aiding in the synthesis of essential vitamins, and extracting nutrients that are otherwise inaccessible from the diet, facilitating the renewal of epithelial cells, regulating fat storage, preserving the integrity of the intestinal barrier, and contributing to brain development [3 - 5]. When it comes to the gut microbiota, research has demonstrated that both vitamin D and the vitamin D receptor (VDR); which serve as mediators for the biological functions of the active form of vitamin D3 [6], are widely distributed throughout the gastrointestinal tract, and have the capacity to influence the composition of the gut microbiota [7]. They play a significant role in immune regulation, cell proliferation, as well as mantaining intestinal equilibrium [8] as shown in Fig. (1).

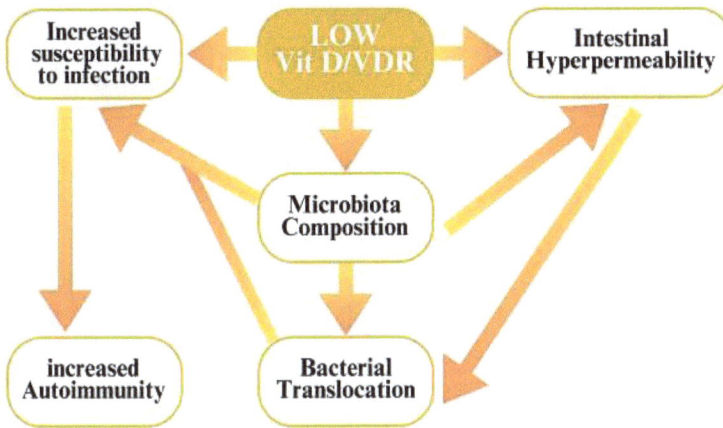

Fig. (1). Relationship of Vitamin D, autoimmunity and gut.

Vitamin D functions as an immune modulator. Notably, it stimulates the production of pattern recognition receptors, antimicrobial peptides, and cytokines, all of which play pivotal roles in initiating innate immune responses. These components are crucial for sensing the presence of the gut microbiota, preventing excessive bacterial overgrowth, and complementing the actions of vitamin D in fortifying the integrity of the intestinal barrier. Additionally, vitamin D promotes the development of tolerogenic T cells, emphasizing a less inflammatory and more immune-tolerant response [9, 10].

Both autoimmune responses and vitamin D, specifically its precursor 25-hydroxyvitamin D (25(OH)D: calcifediol) along with its active form, 1,25-dihydroxyvitamin D (1,25(OH)2D: calcitriol), have essential functions in safeguarding individuals against invading pathogens, decreasing the likelihood of autoimmune disorders, and upholding overall well-being. Conversely, having insufficient levels of 25(OH)D heightens vulnerability to infections and the development of autoimmune conditions [11].

In regard to immune cells, the regulation of both innate and adaptive immunity relies on the precise production of the active form of vitamin D, calcitriol. This process enhances the innate response, marked by the activation of monocytes or macrophages with potent antimicrobial activity [12 - 16]. Additionally, calcitriol promotes the production of immunoglobulin and enhances the stability of B-cells, by influencing B lymphocytes and plasma cells [17, 18], thereby increasing the synthesis of antimicrobial peptides [11].

Furthermore, vitamin D has a broad immunomodulatory effect on innate and adaptive immune responses, it also plays an effective role with T-helper cells, macrophages, and dendritic cells [19, 20]. Calcitriol regulates immunological responses by partially inhibiting B-cell IgE expression and increasing the anti-inflammatory Interleukin-10 expression through dendritic cells and T cells [21 - 23]. In this chapter, we will be adventuring into the benefits of vitamin D with immunity, including autoimmune disorders, the effect of deficiency and sufficiency of vitamin D on immunity and autoimmune disorders, including multiple sclerosis, Hashimoto's Thyroiditis, and rheumatoid arthritis [11].

Gut Microbiota and Vitamin D

The gut microbiome plays a crucial role in human health, influencing the course of chronic illnesses like metabolic diseases, gastrointestinal problems, and colorectal cancer. Environmental factors and dietary patterns significantly impact the establishment of gut microbiota [24 - 26]. In the human gastrointestinal tract (GI tract), approximately 200 common bacteria, viruses, and fungi undertake specific metabolic tasks essential to both health and illness [27 - 29].

The distal gut microbiome is particularly influential in maintaining host health by producing vitamins, essential amino acids, and metabolic byproducts derived from dietary components unabsorbed by the small intestine [30]. Although the gut microbial dynamics in a healthy individual tend to be stable, it is likely that the lifestyle and dietary habits of the host can influence microbial dynamics [25, 31].

A recent systematic review of *in vivo* studies investigated the association between the different levels of vitamin D and Gut Microbiota [32], the study found evidence that suggests a plausible link between vitamin D and the composition of the gastrointestinal microbiome. However, it is important to note that the current research is somewhat constrained as many of the studies have been conducted either in mice or in relatively small, specific human populations [32].

The relationship between dysbiosis and various diseases, including cancer, diabetes, cardiovascular disease, and autoimmune diseases, appears to be mostly based on this latter function [33]. Thus, Vitamin D's ability to alter the microbiota of the gut is important for preserving immune system performance and, by extension, human health [34, 35].

The active form of VD3, widely expressed in the gut, plays a crucial role in immunological modulation, proliferation, and intestinal homeostasis, mediated biologically by VDRs [35]. While the direct impact of vitamin D on bacteria is not fully understood, certain mycobacterial species show inhibited growth when exposed to vitamin D *in vitro*, aligning with its well-known immunoregulatory capabilities [34, 36].

Recent evidence suggests that Vitamin D may have an indirect effect on the gut microbiota composition, consistent with findings from various studies [35, 37, 38]. One mechanism through which Vitamin D can affect microbial composition is the presence of vitamin D receptors at the gastrointestinal level, particularly in controlling the immune response [39]. Additionally, antimicrobial peptides such as cathelicidin and defensin, produced by VDRs, contribute to maintaining microbial equilibrium [19, 40]. Further research suggests that Vitamin D and VDRs have an impact on the regulation and maintenance of gut integrity and the function of microbiota, by suppressing beta-catenin and upregulating the expression of tight junction proteins like ZO-1, Occludin, and E-cadherin [34, 41].

A recent randomized controlled trial examining university students with vitamin D deficiency focusing on improving their health through a 90-day program showed positive outcomes. The group receiving additional treatment, including a combination of probiotics (synbiotic) and vitamin D3, along with guidance on nutrition and physical activity, experienced significant improvements in mental well-being, increased vitamin D levels, and reductions in body weight, body mass index, waist circumference, and fatty mass [42].

A systematic review of human studies investigated the relationship between Vitamin D (VD) and human microbiota composition, involving participants of all ages, both healthy and non-healthy [34]. The study included interventional and observational research, assessing factors such as alpha diversity, beta diversity, species richness, and prevalence of bacterial taxa. Additionally, another systematic review focused on the relationship between Vitamin D and the gastrointestinal microbiome, reviewing mouse and human studies and highlighting the impact of Vitamin D levels and genetic factors on microbiome composition, particularly increasing bacteroidetes in low Vitamin D conditions [32].

In a similar review, numerous research papers have shown a connection between low vitamin D levels and the onset of dysbiosis. Additionally, research on interventions has revealed that vitamin D can alter the microbiome composition by promoting beneficial bacteria and decreasing the Firmicutes/Bacteroides ratio [43].

Hypovitaminosis D and Immunity

Vitamin D regulates autoimmunity by inhibiting adaptive immunity through the suppression of T- and B-lymphocyte activity [44, 45]. Evidence from a systematic review of the health risks of hypovitaminosis reveals that insufficient vitamin D levels (<72.5 nmol/L; <30 ng/ml) impact 50% of the global population, with 1 billion people experiencing vitamin D deficiency (<25 nmol/L; <10 ng/ml) according to the Endocrine Society Clinical Practice Guidelines [46 - 49].

Consequently, hypovitaminosis of vitamin D results in a compromised immune system, serving as a primary trigger for autoimmune responses [49 - 53] as shown in Fig. (**2**). Additionally, individuals with low serum levels of 25(OH)D face exacerbated autoimmune diseases [54, 55], such as multiple sclerosis (MS) [56].

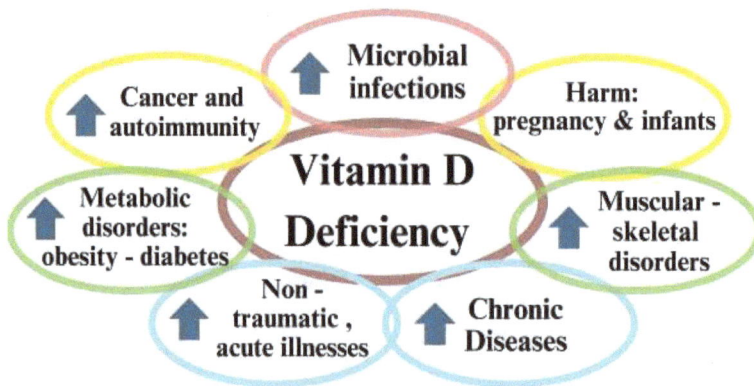

Fig. (2). Vitamin D deficiency and immunity. Adapted with permission form [11].

Insufficient vitamin D levels, also known as Hypovitaminosis D, also heighten the risk of autoimmune diseases [52, 53]. Individuals with various autoimmune disorders, including autoimmune adrenal disease, Multiple Sclerosis (MS), and Hashimoto's thyroiditis, exhibit lower serum levels of 25(OH)D [50, 51, 57].

These findings strongly suggest a negative correlation between vitamin D levels and autoimmunity, meaning that lower concentrations of serum 25(OH)D appear to be associated with increased risks of both the incidence and severity of autoimmune conditions [11, 51 - 53,].

This correlation extends to multiple sclerosis (MS), where a recent review confirmed the impact of Vitamin D on the immune response in MS patients through numerous *in vitro* studies. Additionally, several studies in animal models of MS and experimental autoimmune encephalomyelitis (EAE) strongly indicate the protective role of Vitamin D. Consistently, several studies have verified that levels of 25(OH)D are lower in MS patients, ranging from 20% to 84%, in comparison to healthy controls [58 - 60]. Intriguingly, individuals with progressive forms of MS and increased disability display even lower Vitamin D levels [52, 59, 61].

In the context of autoimmune diseases and Vitamin D deficiency, a recent review has explored the connection between Vitamin D, inflammation, and Hashimoto Thyroiditis (HT), generating interest among researchers globally [52, 62].

Observational studies consistently indicate a higher prevalence of vitamin D deficiency in individuals with HT [63] and suggest an inverse correlation between circulating Vitamin D levels and thyroid antibody levels [64, 65]. However, results remain inconclusive, as some studies show a weak or absent relationship between Vitamin D levels and the Thyroid Peroxidase Antibodies TPOAb titer [66, 67]. Another study obtained conflicting results, noting higher Vitamin D levels in a cohort of HT women compared to female controls [68], but not in men [52].

In a recent study in western Saudi Arabia, a retrospective analysis included 100 rheumatoid arthritis patients and 100 controls, to estimate the prevalence of low serum vitamin D levels (25(OH)D) in RA patients compared to healthy controls. While serum vitamin D levels in RA patients are similar to the healthy control group, significantly lower 25(OH)D values are found in patients with poor treatment response and those not in a state of disease remission [69].

In addition, a case-control study examined the prevalence of Vitamin D and its determinants of deficiency in RA patients compared to healthy controls. The authors concluded that vitamin D deficiency is common in RA patients and comparable to ones found in control subjects [70].

Vitamin D Sufficiency and Immunity

In contrast, maintaining optimal levels of vitamin D in the body is crucial for immune function. Adequate production of calcitriol within immune cells serves a regulatory role in both innate and adaptive immunity, supporting the innate response, especially in monocytes or macrophages that possess antimicrobial activity [12 - 16]. Additionally, calcitriol influences B lymphocytes as well as plasma cells, stimulating immunoglobulin production and providing stability to B-cells [17, 18], thereby increasing the synthesis of anti-microbial peptides [11].

Vitamin D exerts a modulatory effect on various immune cell types, including monocytes/macrophages, dendritic cells, and B and T cells [16]. Fig. (3) shows the effects of vitamin D on different immune cells and the role of each cell. The final result is the regulation of immune response.

DC: Dendritic cell; Ig: Immunoglobulin; IL: Interleukin; MHC: Major histocompatibility complex; IgM: Immunoglobin M; IgG: Immunoglobin G [71].

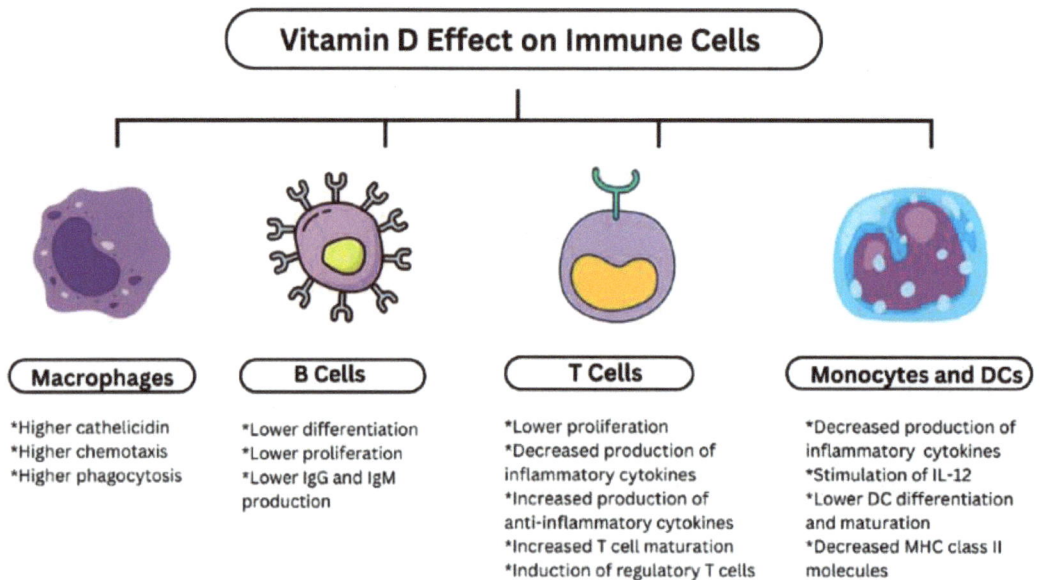

Vitamin D Effect on Immune Cells

Macrophages	B Cells	T Cells	Monocytes and DCs
*Higher cathelicidin *Higher chemotaxis *Higher phagocytosis	*Lower differentiation *Lower proliferation *Lower IgG and IgM production	*Lower proliferation *Decreased production of inflammatory cytokines *Increased production of anti-inflammatory cytokines *Increased T cell maturation *Induction of regulatory T cells	*Decreased production of inflammatory cytokines *Stimulation of IL-12 *Lower DC differentiation and maturation *Decreased MHC class II molecules

Fig. (3). The effects of vitamin D on different immune cells.

Recent evidence from epidemiological, cross-sectional, and longitudinal studies strongly supports the idea that maintaining the serum level of 25(OH)D, at more than 40 ng/mL, significantly diminishes the incidence of extra-musculoskeletal disorders. This encompasses conditions such as diabetes [72], multiple sclerosis (MS) [73], rheumatoid arthritis [74], osteoporosis [75, 76], and autoimmune diseases [77], and contributes to a reduction in all-cause mortality [11, 78].

Sufficiency of vitamin D has been studied in relation to Multiple Sclerosis. In a study by Munger *et al.*, it was revealed that elevated serum levels of 25(OH)D were linked to a substantially lower risk of incident MS, particularly in Caucasians and individuals under 20 years of age, whereas no significant association was observed in Afro-Americans or Hispanics [79]. Additionally, the

same research group found that women consuming more than 400 IUs of vitamin D per day experienced a 41% reduction in the risk of developing MS [52, 73].

Regarding Hashimoto's disease and its relation to Vitamin D sufficiency, recent review studies have delved into the majority of available randomized control trials, which have demonstrated the capacity of Vitamin D (Vit D) to reduce the TPOAb titer [80 - 83]. Krysiak's findings indicated that cholecalciferol effectively lowered TPOAb titers in Hashimoto's thyroiditis (HT) women whose hypothyroidism was well managed with levothyroxine treatment [82].

In a study involving 218 individuals with normal thyroid function (euthyroid) diagnosed with Hashimoto's thyroiditis (HT) and concurrent Vitamin D deficiency, a noteworthy decrease (−20.3%) in thyroid peroxidase antibodies (TPOAb) titer was observed after supplementation with cholecalciferol (1200–4000 IU/day for 4 months) [80]. It is important to note, however, that the influence of Vitamin D supplementation on the recovery from hypothyroidism has not been definitively established [52, 84].

The relationship between vitamin D and rheumatoid arthritis has been explored in numerous studies. In a cohort study focused on arthritis patients, it was observed in regard to serum concentration of 25-hydroxyvitamin D, for every 10-ng/mL increase in its levels, there was a significant decrease in the Disease Activity Score-28. Additionally, this increase in vitamin D levels was associated with a 25% reduction in serum C-reactive protein (CRP) levels. This suggests a potential correlation between higher vitamin D levels and a decrease in both disease activity and inflammation markers in individuals with arthritis [85]. This finding highlights the protective impact of Vitamin D, particularly its active form, as an anti-inflammatory, especially in relation to rheumatoid arthritis [11, 86].

Moreover, individuals with a rare genetic disorder of resistance to calcitriol, exhibit a heightened susceptibility to autoimmune diseases such as rheumatoid arthritis [87]. Consequently, individuals with rheumatoid disorders also experience benefits from the supplementation of vitamin D. A recent systematic review discussed rheumatoid arthritis individuals, with acquired tissue resistance to calcitriol, which might benefit from vitamin D analogs [88]. Furthermore, individuals exposed to sufficient doses of ultraviolet B (UVB) have experienced a reduction in complications and slowed the progression of the autoimmune disease rheumatoid arthritis [11, 18, 89, 90].

A recent study proposed that vitamin D plays an important role in both cancer and immunological regulation. Researchers working with mice found that they have higher vitamin D availability, which show enhanced immune-dependent resistance to malignancies that can be transplanted, as well as enhanced responses to immunotherapies that disrupt checkpoints. In humans, vitamin D-induced genes are likewise correlated with enhanced responses to immune checkpoint inhibitor therapy, as well as with resistance to cancer and longer life rates. The activity of vitamin D on intestinal epithelial cells in mice is responsible for resistance; it modifies the composition of the microbiome in favour of Bacteroides fragilis, which favourably regulates immunity against cancer. Researchers' results point to a hitherto overlooked relationship between immune responses against cancer, microbial commensal populations, and vitamin D. Collectively, these findings underscore the potential role of vitamin D levels as an indicator of cancer immunity and the effectiveness of immunotherapy [91].

Vitamin D and Respiratory Diseases

In recent years, there has been a growing interest in the impact of vitamin D on the severity of chronic respiratory diseases. Various studies have shown how vitamin D deficiency or supplementation can influence risk factors linked to the development of chronic airway inflammatory and infectious respiratory conditions [92]. Table **1** summarizes the results of several studies concerning the prevalence of vitamin D deficiency and supplementation in preventing chronic respiratory diseases, including allergic inflammation, chronic obstructive pulmonary disease (COPD), cystic fibrosis (CF), idiopathic pulmonary fibrosis (IPF), tuberculosis (TB), and COVID-19-related lung diseases.

Table 1. Relation of Vitamin D with Respiratory Diseases [92, 93].

Name of Disease	Pathophysiology	Relation to Vit. D
Asthma	Chronic inflammatory disorder of the airways, is often related to vitamin D deficiency by vitamin D deficiency, which has been linked to an increased risk of asthma and other respiratory diseases.	• Some studies indicate that vitamin D supplementation improves steroid response and reduces levels of asthma-related cytokines. • Low maternal vitamin D intake in children is associated with increased wheezing and potential asthma development. Supplementation in early life might enhance immune responses and lung development, though its impact on asthma control remains uncertain.

(Table 1) cont.....

Name of Disease	Pathophysiology	Relation to Vit. D
Chronic Obstructive Pulmonary Disease (COPD)	Persistent respiratory symptoms and airflow limitation due to airway and/or alveolar abnormalities are usually caused by significant exposure to noxious particles or gases.	• Low vitamin D and increased TNF-α levels are linked to airway obstruction in COPD. Vitamin D modulates TNF-α, a key player in COPD inflammation. • Deficient 25(OH)D levels significantly affect lung function parameters (FEV1 and FVC) in COPD patients. • Some trials show reduced COPD exacerbations and improved FEV1 with vitamin D supplementation, suggesting a correlation with better prognosis.
Cystic fibrosis	Genetic disorder that is caused by mutations in the CFTR gene, which results in the production of thick, sticky mucus in various organs, particularly affecting the respiratory and gastrointestinal systems.	• Clinical trials show that vitamin D supplementation can reduce inflammation, improve lung function, and decrease pulmonary exacerbations in CF patients. • Higher 25(OH)D levels correlate with fewer exacerbations and better lung function (improved FEV1). • The active form of vitamin D (1,25(OH)2D) upregulates genes involved in local lung immunity, exerting anti-inflammatory and antimicrobial effects.
Idiopathic pulmonary fibrosis (IPF)	IPF is a progressive form of interstitial lung disease that is characterized by activated fibroblasts and excessive deposition of extracellular matrix (ECM). Damage to aging alveolar epithelium plays a crucial role in IPF, triggering the secretion of pro-fibrotic factors, leading to irreversible fibrosis and cell senescence.	• In a bleomycin-induced pulmonary fibrosis mouse model, vitamin D treatment reduced the responsiveness of lung fibroblasts to pro-fibrotic stimuli. • Vitamin D supplementation significantly decreased markers of extracellular matrix (ECM) deposition, suggesting a potential anti-fibrotic effect. • Vitamin D is proposed as a promising prognostic and potential therapeutic agent for IPF, although further clinical studies are necessary to confirm its efficacy and safety in human patients.
Tuberculosis	Caused by Mycobacterium tuberculosis and begins with inhalation of infectious droplets. The bacteria invade alveolar macrophages, leading to granuloma formation.	• Observational studies suggest that vitamin D deficiency is common among TB patients, and supplementation has been investigated as a potential adjunct to standard TB therapy. • Clinical trials have shown mixed results regarding the efficacy of vitamin D supplementation in improving TB treatment outcomes, including sputum culture conversion rates.

(Table 1) cont.....

Name of Disease	Pathophysiology	Relation to Vit. D
COVID-19	Caused by the SARS-CoV-2 virus, primarily targets the respiratory system by entering cells through ACE2 receptors in the airways. Triggers an immune response characterized by the release of pro-inflammatory cytokines and chemokines, leading to widespread inflammation.	• vitamin D may enhance the expression of ACE2 receptors, which are implicated in SARS-CoV-2 entry into cells. This modulation could potentially mitigate the severity of lung injury and acute respiratory distress syndrome (ARDS) associated with COVID-19. • Epidemiological studies have also shown correlations between vitamin D deficiency and increased susceptibility to COVID-19 infection and severity, although mixed results from clinical trials suggest a need for further research to establish definitive therapeutic benefits of vitamin D supplementation in COVID-19.

CONCLUSION

Vitamin D plays a key role in the gut health and microbiota, which impacts the human body's immunity. Research clearly shows the beneficial effects of vitamin D concerning autoimmune disorders in its sufficiency and deficiency. Further studies are needed to prove its strong association with autoimmune disorders such as Rheumatoid Arthritis, Hashimoto's Thyroiditis, Multiple Sclerosis, and respiratory diseases, especially when it comes to the supplementation of vitamin D.

REFERENCES

[1]   Quigley EMM. Microbiota-brain-gut axis and neurodegenerative diseases. Curr Neurol Neurosci Rep 2017; 17(12): 94.
        [http://dx.doi.org/10.1007/s11910-017-0802-6] [PMID: 29039142]

[2]   Ogbu D, Xia E, Sun J. Gut instincts: vitamin D/vitamin D receptor and microbiome in neurodevelopment disorders. Open Biol 2020; 10(7): 200063.
        [http://dx.doi.org/10.1098/rsob.200063] [PMID: 32634371]

[3]   Sun J. Dietary vitamin D, vitamin D receptor, and microbiome. Curr Opin Clin Nutr Metab Care 2018; 21(6): 471-4.
        [http://dx.doi.org/10.1097/MCO.0000000000000516] [PMID: 30169457]

[4]   Strandwitz P. Neurotransmitter modulation by the gut microbiota. Brain Res. 2018; 1693(Pt B): 128.

[5]   Abboud M, Rizk R, AlAnouti F, Papandreou D, Haidar S, Mahboub N. The health effects of vitamin d and probiotic co-supplementation: A systematic review of randomized controlled trials. Nutrients 2020; 13(1): 111.
        [http://dx.doi.org/10.3390/nu13010111] [PMID: 33396898]

[6]   Bellerba F, Muzio V, Gnagnarella P, et al. The association between vitamin D and gut microbiota: A systematic review of human studies. Nutrients 2021; 13(10): 3378.
        [http://dx.doi.org/10.3390/nu13103378] [PMID: 34684379]

[7]   Shang M, Sun J. Vitamin D/VDR, probiotics, and gastrointestinal diseases. Curr Med Chem 2017; 24(9): 876-87.
[http://dx.doi.org/10.2174/0929867323666161202150008] [PMID: 27915988]

[8]   Myers SP. The causes of intestinal dysbiosis: A review. Altern Med Rev 2004; x: 9.

[9]   Rawat D, Roy A, Maitra S, Shankar V, Khanna P, Baidya DK. Vitamin D supplementation and COVID-19 treatment: A systematic review and meta-analysis. Diabetes Metab Syndr 2021; 15(4): 102189.
[http://dx.doi.org/10.1016/j.dsx.2021.102189] [PMID: 34217144]

[10]   Dimitrov V, White JH. Vitamin D signaling in intestinal innate immunity and homeostasis. Mol Cell Endocrinol 2017; 453: 68-78.
[http://dx.doi.org/10.1016/j.mce.2017.04.010] [PMID: 28412519]

[11]   Wimalawansa SJ. infections and autoimmunity—the immune system and vitamin D: A systematic review. nutrients. 2023; 15(17).

[12]   Ganmaa D, Enkhmaa D, Nasantogtokh E, Sukhbaatar S, Tumur-Ochir KE, Manson JE. Vitamin D, respiratory infections, and chronic disease: Review of meta-analyses and randomized clinical trials. J Intern Med 2022; 291(2): 141-64.
[http://dx.doi.org/10.1111/joim.13399] [PMID: 34537990]

[13]   Vintilescu BȘ, Niculescu CE, Stepan MD, Ioniță E. Involvement of Vitamin D in chronic infections of the waldeyer's ring in the school aged child. Curr Health Sci J 2019; 45(3): 291-5.
[PMID: 32042457]

[14]   Juszczak AB, Kupczak M, Konecki T. Does vitamin supplementation play a role in chronic kidney disease? Nutrients 2023; 15(13): 2847.
[http://dx.doi.org/10.3390/nu15132847] [PMID: 37447174]

[15]   Özdemir B, Köksal BT, Karakaş NM, Tekindal MA, Özbek ÖY. Serum vitamin D levels in children with recurrent respiratory infections and chronic cough. Indian J Pediatr 2016; 83(8): 777-82.
[http://dx.doi.org/10.1007/s12098-015-2010-1] [PMID: 26821547]

[16]   Song L, Papaioannou G, Zhao H, *et al.* The vitamin D receptor regulates tissue resident macrophage response to injury. Endocrinology 2016; 157(10): 4066-75.
[http://dx.doi.org/10.1210/en.2016-1474] [PMID: 27526034]

[17]   Ao T, Kikuta J, Ishii M. The effects of vitamin D on immune system and inflammatory diseases. Biomolecules 2021; 11(11): 1624.
[http://dx.doi.org/10.3390/biom11111624] [PMID: 34827621]

[18]   Cutolo M, Pizzorni C, Sulli A. Vitamin D endocrine system involvement in autoimmune rheumatic diseases. Autoimmun Rev 2011; 11(2): 84-7.
[http://dx.doi.org/10.1016/j.autrev.2011.08.003] [PMID: 21864722]

[19]   Wang TT, Nestel FP, Bourdeau V, *et al.* Cutting edge: 1,25-dihydroxyvitamin D3 is a direct inducer of antimicrobial peptide gene expression. J Immunol 2004; 173(5): 2909-12.
[http://dx.doi.org/10.4049/jimmunol.173.5.2909] [PMID: 15322146]

[20]   Lin Z, Li W. The roles of vitamin D and its analogs in inflammatory diseases. Curr Top Med Chem 2016; 16(11): 1242-61.
[http://dx.doi.org/10.2174/1568026615666150915111557] [PMID: 26369816]

[21]   Heine G, Niesner U, Chang HD, *et al.* 1,25-dihydroxyvitamin D $_3$ promotes IL-10 production in human B cells. Eur J Immunol 2008; 38(8): 2210-8.
[http://dx.doi.org/10.1002/eji.200838216] [PMID: 18651709]

[22]   Bikle DD. Vitamin D regulation of immune function during covid-19. Rev Endocr Metab Disord 2022; 23(2): 279-85.
[http://dx.doi.org/10.1007/s11154-021-09707-4] [PMID: 35091881]

[23] Vanherwegen AS, Gysemans C, Mathieu C. Regulation of immune function by vitamin D and its use in diseases of immunity. Endocrinol Metab Clin North Am 2017; 46(4): 1061-94.
[http://dx.doi.org/10.1016/j.ecl.2017.07.010] [PMID: 29080635]

[24] Conlon MA, Bird AR. The impact of diet and lifestyle on gut microbiota and human health. nutrients. 2015; 7(1): 17.

[25] Singh RK, Chang HW, Yan D, *et al.* Influence of diet on the gut microbiome and implications for human health. J Transl Med 2017; 15(1): 73.
[http://dx.doi.org/10.1186/s12967-017-1175-y] [PMID: 28388917]

[26] Brennan CA, Garrett WS. Gut microbiota, inflammation, and colorectal cancer. Annu Rev Microbiol 2016; 70(1): 395-411.
[http://dx.doi.org/10.1146/annurev-micro-102215-095513] [PMID: 27607555]

[27] Valdes AM, Walter J, Segal E, Spector TD. Role of the gut microbiota in nutrition and health. BMJ 2018; 361: k2179.
[http://dx.doi.org/10.1136/bmj.k2179] [PMID: 29899036]

[28] Qin J, Li R, Raes J, *et al.* A human gut microbial gene catalogue established by metagenomic sequencing. Nature 2010; 464(7285): 59-65.
[http://dx.doi.org/10.1038/nature08821] [PMID: 20203603]

[29] Hills RD, Pontefract BA, Mishcon HR, Black CA, Sutton SC, Theberge CR. Gut microbiome: Profound implications for diet and disease. Nutrients. 2019; 11(7).

[30] Bäckhed F, Ley RE, Sonnenburg JL, Peterson DA, Gordon JI. Host-bacterial mutualism in the human intestine. Science 2005; 307(5717): 1915-20.
[http://dx.doi.org/10.1126/science.1104816] [PMID: 15790844]

[31] Wu GD, Chen J, Hoffmann C, *et al.* Linking long-term dietary patterns with gut microbial enterotypes. Science 2011; 334(6052): 105-8.
[http://dx.doi.org/10.1126/science.1208344] [PMID: 21885731]

[32] Waterhouse M, Hope B, Krause L, *et al.* Vitamin D and the gut microbiome: a systematic review of *in vivo* studies. Eur J Nutr 2019; 58(7): 2895-910.
[http://dx.doi.org/10.1007/s00394-018-1842-7] [PMID: 30324342]

[33] Rinninella E, Raoul P, Cintoni M, *et al.* What is the healthy gut microbiota composition? a changing ecosystem across age, environment, Diet, and Diseases. Microorganisms 2019; 7(1): 14.
[http://dx.doi.org/10.3390/microorganisms7010014] [PMID: 30634578]

[34] Bellerba F, Muzio V, Gnagnarella P, *et al.* The association between Vitamin D and gut microbiota: A systematic review of human studies. Nutrients. 2021; 13(10).

[35] Fakhoury HMA, Kvietys PR, AlKattan W, *et al.* Vitamin D and intestinal homeostasis: Barrier, microbiota, and immune modulation. J Steroid Biochem Mol Biol 2020; 200: 105663.
[http://dx.doi.org/10.1016/j.jsbmb.2020.105663] [PMID: 32194242]

[36] Greenstein RJ, Su L, Brown ST, Vitamins A. Vitamins A & D inhibit the growth of mycobacteria in radiometric culture. PLoS One 2012; 7(1): e29631.
[http://dx.doi.org/10.1371/journal.pone.0029631] [PMID: 22235314]

[37] Malaguarnera L. Vitamin D and microbiota: Two sides of the same coin in the immunomodulatory aspects. Int Immunopharmacol 2020; 79: 106112.
[http://dx.doi.org/10.1016/j.intimp.2019.106112] [PMID: 31877495]

[38] Yamamoto EA, Jørgensen TN. Relationships Between Vitamin D, Gut Microbiome, and Systemic Autoimmunity. Front Immunol 2020; 10: 3141.
[http://dx.doi.org/10.3389/fimmu.2019.03141] [PMID: 32038645]

[39] Bakke D, Sun J. Ancient nuclear receptor vdr with new functions: microbiome and inflammation. Inflamm Bowel Dis 2018; 24(6): 1149-54.

[http://dx.doi.org/10.1093/ibd/izy092] [PMID: 29718408]

[40]   Gombart AF, Borregaard N, Koeffler HP. Human cathelicidin antimicrobial peptide (CAMP) gene is a direct target of the vitamin D receptor and is strongly up-regulated in myeloid cells by 1,25-dihydroxyvitamin D $_3$. FASEB J 2005; 19(9): 1067-77.
[http://dx.doi.org/10.1096/fj.04-3284com] [PMID: 15985530]

[41]   Zhang Y, Wu S, Sun J. Vitamin D, vitamin D receptor and tissue barriers. Tissue Barriers 2013; 1(1): e23118.
[http://dx.doi.org/10.4161/tisb.23118] [PMID: 24358453]

[42]   Tokarchuk A, Abenavoli L, Kobyliak N, *et al.* Nutrition program, physical activity and gut microbiota modulation: a randomized controlled trial to promote a healthy lifestyle in students with vitamin D3 deficiency. Minerva Med 2022; 113(4): 683-94.
[http://dx.doi.org/10.23736/S0026-4806.22.07992-7] [PMID: 35912804]

[43]   Aggeletopoulou I, Tsounis EP, Mouzaki A, Triantos C. Exploring the role of vitamin d and the vitamin d receptor in the composition of the gut microbiota. Front Biosci (Landmark Ed). 2023 Jun 14; 28(6): 116.
[http://dx.doi.org/10.31083/j.fbl2806116] [PMID: 37395032]

[44]   Giannini S, Giusti A, Minisola S, Napoli N, Passeri G, Rossini M, Sinigaglia L. The immunologic profile of vitamin d and its role in different immune-mediated diseases: an expert opinion. Nutrients. 2022 Jan 21; 14(3): 473.
[http://dx.doi.org/10.3390/nu14030473] [PMID: 35276834] [PMCID: PMC8838062]

[45]   Wimalawansa SJ. Infections and autoimmunity—the immune system and vitamin D: A systematic review. Nutrients. 2023; 15(17).

[46]   Hoseinzadeh E, Taha P, Wei C, *et al.* The impact of air pollutants, UV exposure and geographic location on vitamin D deficiency. Food Chem Toxicol 2018; 113: 241-54.
[http://dx.doi.org/10.1016/j.fct.2018.01.052] [PMID: 29409825]

[47]   Lucas RM, Gorman S, Black L, Neale RE. Clinical, research, and public health implications of poor measurement of vitamin D status. J AOAC Int 2017; 100(5): 1225-9.
[http://dx.doi.org/10.5740/jaoacint.17-0082] [PMID: 28492144]

[48]   Schramm S, Lahner H, Jöckel KH, Erbel R, Führer D, Moebus S. Impact of season and different vitamin D thresholds on prevalence of vitamin D deficiency in epidemiological cohorts—a note of caution. Endocrine 2017; 56(3): 658-66.
[http://dx.doi.org/10.1007/s12020-017-1292-7] [PMID: 28417313]

[49]   Caccamo D, Ricca S, Currò M, Ientile R. Health risks of hypovitaminosis d: a review of new molecular insights. Int J Mol Sci 2018; 19(3): 892.
[http://dx.doi.org/10.3390/ijms19030892] [PMID: 29562608]

[50]   Delvin E, Souberbielle JC, Viard JP, Salle B. Role of vitamin D in acquired immune and autoimmune diseases. Crit Rev Clin Lab Sci 2014; 51(4): 232-47.
[http://dx.doi.org/10.3109/10408363.2014.901291] [PMID: 24813330]

[51]   Sîrbe C, Rednic S, Grama A, Pop TL. An update on the effects of vitamin D on the immune system and autoimmune diseases. Int J Mol Sci 2022; 23(17): 9784.
[http://dx.doi.org/10.3390/ijms23179784] [PMID: 36077185]

[52]   Gallo D, Baci D, Kustrimovic N, *et al.* How does vitamin D affect immune cells crosstalk in autoimmune diseases? Int J Mol Sci 2023; 24(5): 4689.
[http://dx.doi.org/10.3390/ijms24054689] [PMID: 36902117]

[53]   Székely JI, Pataki Á. Effects of vitamin D on immune disorders with special regard to asthma, COPD and autoimmune diseases: a short review. Expert Rev Respir Med 2012; 6(6): 683-704.
[http://dx.doi.org/10.1586/ers.12.57] [PMID: 23234453]

[54]   Hassan V, Hassan S, Seyed-Javad P, *et al.* Association between serum 25 (OH) vitamin D

concentrations and inflammatory bowel diseases (IBDs) Activity.

[55]   Sainaghi PP, Bellan M, Nerviani A, *et al.* Superiority of a high loading dose of cholecalciferol to correct hypovitaminosis d in patients with inflammatory/autoimmune rheumatic diseases. J Rheumatol 2013; 40(2): 166-72.
[http://dx.doi.org/10.3899/jrheum.120536] [PMID: 23242183]

[56]   Tuohimaa P, Keisala T, Minasyan A, Cachat J, Kalueff A. Vitamin D, nervous system and aging. Psychoneuroendocrinology. 2009; 34(1).

[57]   Pani MA, Regulla K, Segni M, *et al.* Vitamin D 1alpha-hydroxylase (CYP1alpha) polymorphism in Graves' disease, Hashimoto's thyroiditis and type 1 diabetes mellitus. Eur J Endocrinol 2002; 146(6): 777-81.
[http://dx.doi.org/10.1530/eje.0.1460777] [PMID: 12039697]

[58]   Kragt JJ, van Amerongen BM, Killestein J, *et al.* Higher levels of 25-hydroxyvitamin D are associated with a lower incidence of multiple sclerosis only in women. Mult Scler 2009; 15(1): 9-15.
[http://dx.doi.org/10.1177/1352458508095920] [PMID: 18701572]

[59]   Smolders J, Menheere P, Kessels A, Damoiseaux J, Hupperts R. Association of vitamin D metabolite levels with relapse rate and disability in multiple sclerosis. 2008; 14(9): 1220–4.
[http://dx.doi.org/10.1177/1352458508094399]

[60]   Hiremath GS, Cettomai D, Baynes M, *et al.* Vitamin D status and effect of low-dose cholecalciferol and high-dose ergocalciferol supplementation in multiple sclerosis. 2009; 15(6): 735–40.
[http://dx.doi.org/10.1177/1352458509102844]

[61]   Correale J, Ysrraelit MC, Gaitán MI. Immunomodulatory effects of Vitamin D in multiple sclerosis. Brain 2009; 132(5): 1146-60.
[http://dx.doi.org/10.1093/brain/awp033] [PMID: 19321461]

[62]   Xu MY, Cao B, Yin J, Wang DF, Chen KL, Lu Q Bin. Vitamin D and graves' disease: A meta-analysis update. Nutrients, 2015; 7(5): 3813–27.

[63]   Kim D. Low vitamin D status is associated with hypothyroid Hashimoto's thyroiditis. Hormones (Athens) 2016; 15(3): 385-93.
[http://dx.doi.org/10.14310/horm.2002.1681] [PMID: 27394703]

[64]   Wang X, Zynat J, Guo Y, *et al.* Low serum vitamin D is associated with anti-thyroid-globulin antibody in female individuals. Int J Endocrinol. 2015; 2015.

[65]   Mukhopadhyay S, Chaudhary S, Dutta D, *et al.* Vitamin D supplementation reduces thyroid peroxidase antibody levels in patients with autoimmune thyroid disease: An open-labeled randomized controlled trial. Indian J Endocrinol Metab 2016; 20(3): 391-8.
[http://dx.doi.org/10.4103/2230-8210.179997] [PMID: 27186560]

[66]   Goswami R, Marwaha RK, Gupta N, *et al.* Prevalence of vitamin D deficiency and its relationship with thyroid autoimmunity in Asian Indians: a community-based survey. Br J Nutr 2009; 102(3): 382-6.https://www.cambridge.org/core/journals/british-journal-of-nutrition/article/prevalence-of-vi-amin-d-deficiency-and-its-relationship-with-thyroid-autoimmunity-in-asi-n-indians-a-communitybased-survey/1E9AEC423D2594B020BC54551E98CA6E
[http://dx.doi.org/10.1017/S0007114509220824] [PMID: 19203420]

[67]   Ke W, Sun T, Zhang Y, *et al.* 25-Hydroxyvitamin D serum level in Hashimoto's thyroiditis, but not Graves' disease is relatively deficient. Endocr J 2017; 64(6): 581-7.
[http://dx.doi.org/10.1507/endocrj.EJ16-0547] [PMID: 28413173]

[68]   Yasmeh J, Farpour F, Rizzo V, Kheradnam S, Sachmechi I. Hashimoto thyroiditis not associated with Vitamin D deficiency. Endocr Pract 2016; 22(7): 809-13.
[http://dx.doi.org/10.4158/EP15934.OR] [PMID: 27018618]

[69]   Alharbi S, Alharbi R, Alhabib E, Ghunaim R, Alreefi MM, Vitamin D. Vitamin D deficiency in saudi patients with rheumatoid arthritis. Cureus 2023; 15(2): e34815.

[http://dx.doi.org/10.7759/cureus.34815] [PMID: 36793500]

[70] Rossini M, Maddali Bongi S, La Montagna G, *et al.* Vitamin D deficiency in rheumatoid arthritis: prevalence, determinants and associations with disease activity and disability. Arthritis Res Ther 2010; 12(6): R216.
[http://dx.doi.org/10.1186/ar3195] [PMID: 21114806]

[71] Vassiliou AG, Jahaj E, Orfanos SE, Dimopoulou I, Kotanidou A. Vitamin D in infectious complications in critically ill patients with or without COVID-19. Metabolism Open 2021; 11: 100106.
[http://dx.doi.org/10.1016/j.metop.2021.100106] [PMID: 34250458]

[72] Chiu KC, Chu A, Go VLW, Saad MF. Hypovitaminosis D is associated with insulin resistance and β cell dysfunction. Am J Clin Nutr 2004; 79(5): 820-5.
[http://dx.doi.org/10.1093/ajcn/79.5.820] [PMID: 15113720]

[73] Munger KL, Zhang SM, O'Reilly E, *et al.* Vitamin D intake and incidence of multiple sclerosis. Neurology 2004; 62(1): 60-5.
[http://dx.doi.org/10.1212/01.WNL.0000101723.79681.38] [PMID: 14718698]

[74] Merlino LA, Curtis J, Mikuls TR, Cerhan JR, Criswell LA, Saag KG. Vitamin D intake is inversely associated with rheumatoid arthritis: Results from the Iowa Women's health study. Arthritis Rheum 2004; 50(1): 72-7.
[http://dx.doi.org/10.1002/art.11434] [PMID: 14730601]

[75] Feskanich D, Willett WC, Colditz GA. Calcium, vitamin D, milk consumption, and hip fractures: a prospective study among postmenopausal women. Am J Clin Nutr 2003; 77(2): 504-11.
[http://dx.doi.org/10.1093/ajcn/77.2.504] [PMID: 12540414]

[76] Meier C, Woitge HW, Witte K, Lemmer B, Seibel MJ. Supplementation with oral vitamin D3 and calcium during winter prevents seasonal bone loss: a randomized controlled open-label prospective trial. J Bone Miner Res 2004; 19(8): 1221-30.
[http://dx.doi.org/10.1359/JBMR.040511] [PMID: 15231008]

[77] Akdere G, Efe B, Sisman P, Yorulmaz G. The relationship between vitamin D level and organ-specific autoimmune disorders in newly diagnosed type I diabetes mellitus. Bratisl Med J 2018; 119(9): 544-9.
[http://dx.doi.org/10.4149/BLL_2018_098] [PMID: 30226063]

[78] Garland CF, Kim JJ, Mohr SB, *et al.* Meta-analysis of all-cause mortality according to serum 25-Hydroxyvitamin D. Am J Public Health. 2014; 104(8): e43.

[79] Munger KL, Levin LI, Hollis BW, Howard NS, Ascherio A. Serum 25-hydroxyvitamin D levels and risk of multiple sclerosis. JAMA 2006; 296(23): 2832-8.
[http://dx.doi.org/10.1001/jama.296.23.2832] [PMID: 17179460]

[80] Gallo D, Mortara L, Gariboldi MB, *et al.* Immunomodulatory effect of vitamin D and its potential role in the prevention and treatment of thyroid autoimmunity: A narrative review. J Endocrinol Invest 2020; 43(4): 413-29.
[http://dx.doi.org/10.1007/s40618-019-01123-5] [PMID: 31584143]

[81] Botelho IMB, Moura Neto A, Silva CA, Tambascia MA, Alegre SM, Zantut-Wittmann DE. Vitamin D in Hashimoto's thyroiditis and its relationship with thyroid function and inflammatory status. Endocr J 2018; 65(10): 1029-37.
[http://dx.doi.org/10.1507/endocrj.EJ18-0166] [PMID: 30058600]

[82] Krysiak R, Szkróbka W, Okopień B. The Effect of Vitamin D on thyroid autoimmunity in levothyroxine-treated women with hashimoto's thyroiditis and normal vitamin D status. Exp Clin Endocrinol Diabetes 2017; 125(4): 229-33.
[http://dx.doi.org/10.1055/s-0042-123038] [PMID: 28073128]

[83] Knutsen KV, Madar AA, Brekke M, *et al.* Effect of vitamin D on thyroid autoimmunity: A randomized, double-blind, controlled trial among ethnic minorities. J Endocr Soc 2017; 1(5): 470-9.

[http://dx.doi.org/10.1210/js.2017-00037] [PMID: 29264502]

[84] Jiang H, Chen X, Qian X, Shao S. Effects of vitamin D treatment on thyroid function and autoimmunity markers in patients with Hashimoto's thyroiditis—A meta-analysis of randomized controlled trials. J Clin Pharm Ther 2022; 47(6): 767-75.
[http://dx.doi.org/10.1111/jcpt.13605] [PMID: 34981556]

[85] Patel S, Farragher T, Berry J, Bunn D, Silman A, Symmons D. Association between serum vitamin D metabolite levels and disease activity in patients with early inflammatory polyarthritis. Arthritis Rheum 2007; 56(7): 2143-9.
[http://dx.doi.org/10.1002/art.22722] [PMID: 17599737]

[86] Jeffery LE, Raza K, Hewison M. Vitamin D in rheumatoid arthritis—towards clinical application. Nat Rev Rheumatol 2016; 12(4): 201-10.
[http://dx.doi.org/10.1038/nrrheum.2015.140] [PMID: 26481434]

[87] Reynolds JA, Bruce IN. Vitamin D treatment for connective tissue diseases: hope beyond the hype? Rheumatology (Oxford) 2017; 56(2): 178-86.
[http://dx.doi.org/10.1093/rheumatology/kew212] [PMID: 27179106]

[88] Tamblyn JA, Hewison M, Wagner CL, Bulmer JN, Kilby MD. Immunological role of vitamin D at the maternal–fetal interface. J Endocrinol 2015; 224(3): R107-21.
[http://dx.doi.org/10.1530/JOE-14-0642] [PMID: 25663707]

[89] Birmingham DJ, Hebert LA, Song H, *et al.* Evidence that abnormally large seasonal declines in vitamin D status may trigger SLE flare in non-African Americans. Lupus 2012; 21(8): 855-64.
[http://dx.doi.org/10.1177/0961203312439640] [PMID: 22433915]

[90] Cutolo M, Otsa K, Laas K, *et al.* Circannual vitamin D serum levels and disease activity in rheumatoid arthritis: Northern versus Southern Europe. Clin Exp Rheumatol 2006; 24(6): 702-4.
[PMID: 17207389]

[91] Giampazolias E, Pereira da Costa M, Lam KC, *et al.* Vitamin D regulates microbiome-dependent cancer immunity. Science 2024; 384(6694): 428-37.
[http://dx.doi.org/10.1126/science.adh7954] [PMID: 38662827]

[92] Gaudet M, Plesa M, Mogas A, Jalaleddine N, Hamid Q, Al Heialy S. Recent advances in vitamin D implications in chronic respiratory diseases. Respiratory Research 2022 23:1. 2022; 23(1)1–14.
[http://dx.doi.org/10.1186/s12931-022-02147-x]

[93] Ismailova A, White JH. Vitamin D, infections and immunity. Rev Endocr Metab Disord 2022; 23(2): 265-77.
[http://dx.doi.org/10.1007/s11154-021-09679-5] [PMID: 34322844]

CHAPTER 3

Vitamin D and Insulin Resistance

Anam Shakil Kalsekar[1,*], **Amina Afrin**[1], **Khawla Jalal**[1] and **Dimitrios Papandreou**[1]

[1] *Department of Clinical Nutrition and Dietetics, College of Health Sciences, University of Sharjah, Sharjah, UAE*

Abstract: This chapter examines the latest research findings on the association between vitamin D levels and insulin resistance (IR) in various populations, including pregnant and postpartum women, children and adolescents, and individuals with certain health conditions such as diabetes, obesity, multiple sclerosis (MS), polycystic ovary syndrome (PCOS), non-alcoholic fatty liver disease (NAFLD), diabetic kidney disease (DKD), and diabetic peripheral neuropathy (DPN). Existing evidence suggests that Vitamin D plays a crucial role as an immunomodulator, affecting important human disorders like insulin resistance, glucose homeostasis, and mineral and bone metabolism. Extensive evidence suggests that vitamin D has a substantial impact on the development of insulin resistance (IR), through its influence on different gene variants related to vitamin D and the metabolic and immunological pathways associated with it. Supplementing with vitamin D can be beneficial in properly managing and enhancing insulin resistance. Diverse research approaches have yielded both favorable and unfavorable results on the correlation between vitamin D and insulin resistance (IR). Further research is recommended to clarify the correlation between vitamin D and insulin function, as well as to determine any variations in this association among different age groups, genders, and illnesses.

Keywords: Diabetes mellitus, Insulin resistance, Metabolic syndrome, Non-Alcoholic fatty liver disease, Vitamin D.

INTRODUCTION

Insulin is a peptide hormone (protein) produced by the beta cells of the pancreatic Langerhans islets. It is the primary anabolic hormone in the human body [1]. This hormone controls the metabolism of all dietary fuels, including carbohydrates, lipids, and proteins. It accelerates postprandial glucose absorption into hepatocytes, lipocytes, and skeletal myocytes for metabolism [1].

* **Corresponding author Anam Shakil Kalsekar:** Department of Clinical Nutrition and Dietetics, College of Health Sciences, University of Sharjah, Sharjah, UAE; E-mails: U23102372@sharjah.ac.ae, anamkalsekar@yahoo.com

Dimitrios Papandreou (Ed.)

As depicted in Fig. (**1**), insulin receptors are present within the cellular membranes. As a first messenger, the hormone insulin initiates a cascade of reactions when it binds to the receptor subunit. In response, myocytes and lipocytes express and insert GLUT4, and the liver and skeletal muscle tissues synthesize glycogen. GLUT4 are the primary transporter proteins involved in glucose metabolism that are activated by insulin [1].

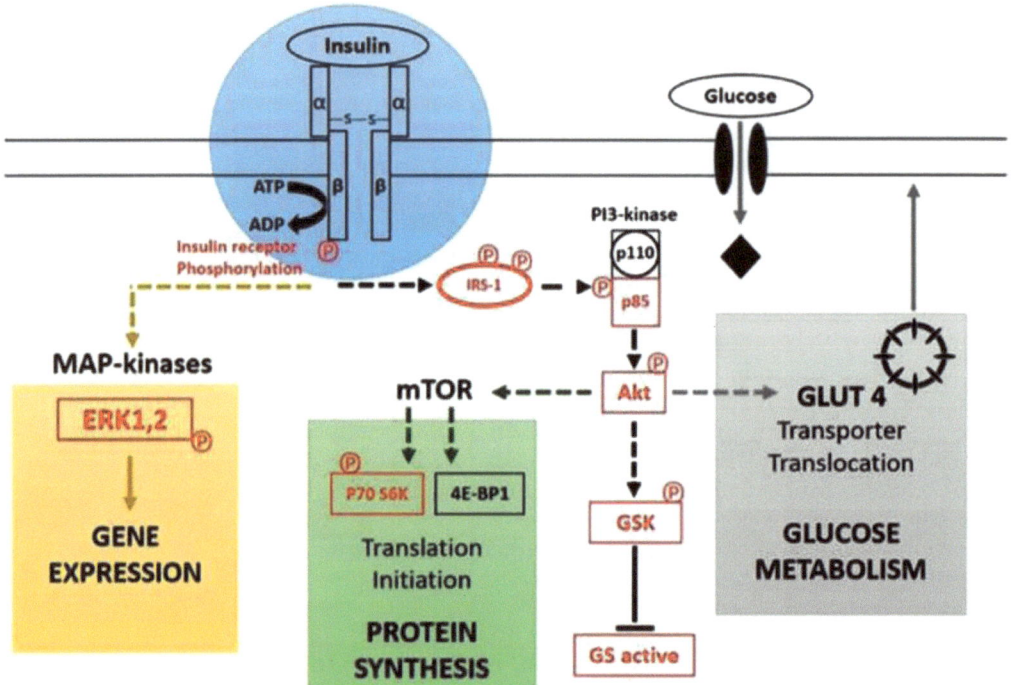

Fig. (1). Insulin signal transduction. The insulin receptor (IR) is in blue, and glucose metabolism (highlighted in grey) [1].

Insulin resistance (IR) is characterized by impaired physiological responses to insulin stimulation in certain target organs, such as the liver, muscle, and adipose tissue. It decreases the efficacy of glucose metabolism, which leads to an increase in insulin synthesis by beta cells and insulin levels [2]. As reported by the National Health and Nutrition Examination Survey (NHANES) conducted in 2021, it was found that over 40% of adults between the ages of 18 and 44 in the United States exhibited IR [2]. Various variables can contribute to the development of the condition, such as age, gender, lack of physical exercise, a significant amount of visceral fat, abdominal obesity, oxidative stress, and mitochondrial dysfunction [3]. Hyperglycemia, hypertension, dyslipidemia, hyperuricemia, elevated inflammatory markers, impaired endothelium function, and a prothrombotic state can result from IR [2].

Comprehending the pathophysiology of IR necessitates the examination of intricate mechanisms that underpin this physiological state. It involves multiple factors and mechanisms, and the key pathophysiological aspects of IR include genetic predisposition, obesity, inflammation, dyslipidemia, adipokines and hormones, insulin signaling pathway, intracellular mechanisms, mitochondrial dysfunction, and feedback mechanisms [4]. Obesity is one of the primary risk factors for IR, which is caused by the overproduction of lipids in adipose tissue, leading to dysfunction [4]. Nevertheless, it is important to note that the issue of IR cannot be only attributed to obesity, as evidenced by the fact that many individuals with prediabetes in various countries are not classified as overweight or obese [1]. Several alternative ideas have been put forth by Aedh *et al.* [1] to provide further understanding of the biology of IR. Among these, an established correlation that has been well-documented in the literature is the strong connection between vitamin D and IR [5]. Vitamin D is classified as a steroid hormone that exerts its physiological effects through interacting with vitamin D receptors (VDRs), a part of the steroid/thyroid receptor family. Similar to insulin receptors, vitamin D receptors (VDRs) are expressed widely throughout the body. Vitamin-receptor binding translocates the complex from the cytosol to the nucleus, where it interacts with retinoid x receptors (RXR). VDR/RXR heterodimers attach to the vitamin D response element (VDRE) in the nucleus, modulating target gene transcription [5]. According to Trimarco *et al.* [5], the expression of about 200 genes is modulated by vitamin D, either upregulated or downregulated. Previous research has indicated that insufficient vitamin D levels might be regarded as either a direct or indirect outcome of IR [5].

Therefore, while the influence of genetic variables on the development and susceptibility of this morbidity is often significant, the impact of environmental events that trigger this morbidity can be substantial. During the initial phases of IR, it is feasible to impede the advancement of the pathological condition. According to Aedh *et al.* [1], oral hypoglycemic medications are the primary therapeutic approach for managing insulin resistance. The specifics pertaining to these agents are beyond the focus of this chapter and, hence, will not be covered. In addition to oral hypoglycemic drugs, research has shown that IR can be treated with methods that control the amount of insulin the body requires, such as dietary and lifestyle modifications [6]. Restoring vitamin D levels in individuals has been shown to efficiently restore insulin sensitivity and perhaps improve IR [5].

A multitude of observational studies have consistently shown a substantial inverse correlation between low levels of serum 25(OH)D and the presence of diabetes, prediabetes, obesity, and metabolic syndrome. As depicted in Fig. (**2**), Trimarco *et al.* [5] observed an inverse relationship between IR and vitamin D levels. This correlation has been linked to an increased vulnerability to a range of disorders. In a similar vein, previous research conducted on animals has shown that the administration of vitamin D (VD) supplements leads to a reduction in IR. This effect is believed to be mediated by the impact of VD on calcium and phosphorus metabolism, as well as the upregulation of the insulin receptor gene [1]. According to the results of a study conducted in Canada, individuals with an increased vulnerability to diabetes or recently diagnosed with T2D demonstrated significant improvements in peripheral insulin sensitivity and β-cell activity after undergoing a six-month regimen of vitamin D supplementation. The study conducted by Lemieux *et al.* [7] suggests that vitamin D might have the capacity to slow down metabolic decline in this particular population.

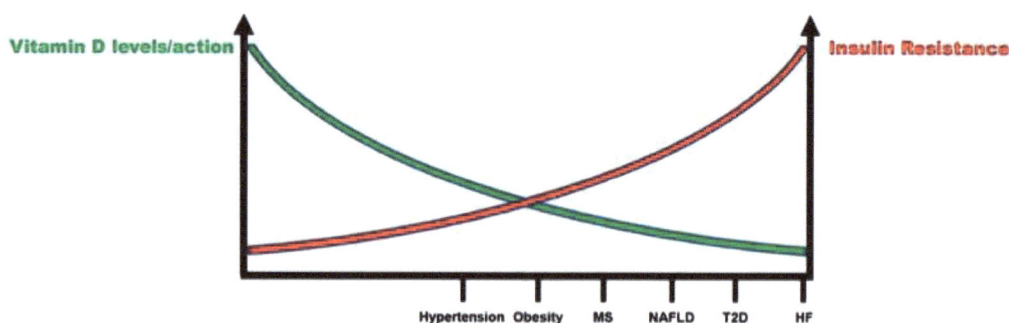

Vitamin D levels/action

Insulin Resistance

Hypertension Obesity MS NAFLD T2D HF

Fig. (2). Correlation between vitamin D status and IR in regards to Metabolic syndrome; Non-alcoholic fatty liver disease; Type 2 diabetes; HF-Heart failure [5].

Moreover, a notable investigation carried out by Aedh *et al.* [1] scrutinized a cohort of 5677 patients exhibiting decreased glucose tolerance. The results of this study indicate that the provision of vitamin D supplements led to a significant improvement in insulin sensitivity, as evidenced by an observed rise of 54%. According to Contreras-Bolívar *et al.* [8], there is evidence suggesting that the higher intake of vitamin D can improve insulin sensitivity.

The following chapter will discuss the most recent body of evidence regarding the association between vitamin D status and IR in pregnant and postpartum women, children and adolescents, and individuals with other comorbidities, such as diabetes, obesity, MS, polycystic ovary syndrome (PCOS), NAFLD, diabetic kidney disease (DKD) and diabetic peripheral neuropathy (DPN). Through the analysis of these studies, our objective is to clarify the potential impact of vitamin D on the management of IR.

Association of Status of Vitamin D and Insulin Resistance in Pregnant and Postpartum Women

This section of the chapter discusses the association between the status of vitamin D and IR in pregnant and postpartum women. Regarding the impact of vitamin D on IR in pregnant and postpartum women, a meta-analysis by Sharafi *et al.* [9] was conducted to assess the impact of vitamin D supplementation on the levels of the homeostatic model of insulin resistance (HOMA-IR) in pregnant women without diabetes. Four studies, comprising a total of six trials and involving 380 participants, provided evidence that vitamin D supplementation leads to a reduction in HOMA-IR levels (mean change: 1.46, 95% CI: 0.56-2.37) when compared to the placebo group. According to Sharafi *et al.* [9], the administration of a high weekly dosage of vitamin D resulted in a significant decline in HOMA-IR levels (p=0.047).

Another research study examined the correlation between vitamin D levels during the middle stage of pregnancy and the development of glucose intolerance after childbirth in women diagnosed with gestational diabetes mellitus (GDM) [10]. The findings of the study indicated that there was a greater occurrence of postpartum glucose intolerance among women who had insufficient levels of vitamin D compared to those who had sufficient levels (48.7% vs. 32.1%, P=0.011). Furthermore, there was an inverse correlation observed between vitamin D levels and HbA1c during both the antepartum and postpartum periods. According to Kim *et al.* [10], women who had a deficiency in vitamin D had a 2.55% greater likelihood of developing postpartum glucose intolerance compared to those who did not have a deficiency (P=0.018; 95% CI: 1.13 to 3.55).

In addition, a prospective longitudinal study was undertaken to investigate the association between IR and vitamin D deficiency in pregnant women [11]. A substantial correlation was found between persistently low levels of vitamin D and increased levels of insulin. Findings of a raw study reported that pregnant women who experience vitamin D insufficiency in the second or third trimester face a 1.83-fold higher likelihood of developing IR [11].

Association of Status of Vitamin D and Insulin Resistance in Children and Adolescents

The following section of the chapter discusses the association of the status of Vitamin D and IR in children and adolescents. Vitamin D deficiency is a significant nutritional concern due to its high prevalence among children [12]. The decrease in blood vitamin D levels can be attributed to several factors, including inadequate dietary intake of vitamin D, reduced outdoor physical activity leading to decreased sun exposure, and a higher proportion of adipose tissue that can sequester vitamin D. There is a positive correlation between insulin sensitivity and circulating 25-OHD. Consequently, deficiencies in glucose metabolism are more probable among obese adolescents who are also deficient in vitamin D [13].

Corsello *et al.* [13] conducted systematic reviews and meta-analyses to evaluate the influence of vitamin D supplementation on metabolic and cardiovascular outcomes in overweight or obese children and adolescents. A cohort of 1959 individuals exhibiting favourable health circumstances was encompassed within 23 studies. The researchers directed their attention to interventional trials that examined the outcome of vitamin D supplementation on children and adolescents who exhibited obesity or overweight conditions. The researches incorporated in this analysis were conducted in multiple countries, encompassing 11 investigations in the United States of America (USA), 3 studies in Iran, two studies in India, and one study each in Finland, France, Greece, Italy, Korea, Poland, and Sri Lanka. The study's exclusion criteria encompassed research that involved participants who were less than 1 year old, as well as studies with a sample size of less than 15 people and individuals with acute or chronic illnesses. Different doses and regimens of vitamin D delivery were tested. A total of 16 investigations implemented a daily regimen of vitamin D, whilst additional studies investigated the impacts of weekly, monthly, or singular administrations. With the exclusion of one particular study, all studies that implemented an average dosage of vitamin D exceeding 20,000 IU per week observed a notable increase in vitamin D levels in persons who were obese.

Among them, a total of 13 studies were undertaken to examine insulin sensitivity and resistance, fasting levels of circulating insulin, and the HOMA-IR index. Among the studies analyzed, six of them documented a beneficial impact of vitamin D supplementation on fasting insulin and HOMA-IR. These effects included a decrease in insulin levels, a reduction in glucose levels, and an improvement in insulin sensitivity. All 6 investigations that were done followed a randomized controlled trial (RCT) design, except for 1 research which utilized a single-arm trial design. The period of the research ranges from a minimum of 12 weeks to a maximum of 6 months. Moreover, there was variation in the dosage of vitamin D among the several investigations. The results suggest a positive association between decreased insulin levels, lowered glucose levels, and improved insulin sensitivity [14 - 19]. In contrast, the metabolic impact of vitamin D was not shown to be statistically significant in 7 studies examining glucose and insulin levels [20 - 26].

Additionally, Corsello *et al.* [13] conducted an extensive inquiry comprising a compilation of 7 meta-analyses, with a specific emphasis on randomized and placebo-controlled studies only. The primary emphasis of the analysis was on clinical trials that evaluated the mean levels of 25-hydroxyvitamin D (25(OH)D) at the beginning and end of the intervention. There was no statistically significant disparity in the average vitamin D levels between the treatment group and the placebo group. Following the successful completion of the intervention, the results demonstrated a statistically significant discrepancy in average values, indicating a mean discrepancy of 1.6 ng/ml between participants who received vitamin D treatment and those who were given a placebo. Nevertheless, the aforementioned inquiries failed to sufficiently investigate or analyze the metabolic repercussions following the intervention, particularly in relation to IR. This study encompasses a contemporary systematic review and meta-analysis that investigates the impact of vitamin D supplementation on children and adolescents who are categorized as overweight or obese. The administration of vitamin D supplements has been observed to result in a substantial increase in concentrations of 25-hydroxyvitamin D (25-OHD). Nevertheless, the assessment of metabolic and cardiovascular outcomes remains a topic of debate due to varying interpretations. Maintaining an optimal amount of Vitamin D is vital for individuals spanning from adolescence to old age, since it is crucial for promoting overall health and well-being. According to Mehmood and Papandreou [27], there is a decrease in blood Vitamin D levels during the onset of puberty. This reduction in Vitamin D levels is associated with an increased risk of obesity. Furthermore, pre-pubertal children with suboptimal serum Vitamin D levels are at a significantly higher risk of developing IR.

Association of Status of Vitamin D and Insulin Resistance in Various Other Diseases

This section of the chapter examines the correlation between Vitamin D status and IR in several other diseases, including obesity, diabetes, MS, PCOS, NAFLD, DKD, and DPN.

Obesity

The increasing prevalence of obesity is a significant health concern associated with Vitamin D. According to the World Health Organization, the global prevalence of overweight adults exceeded 1.9 billion individuals in the year 2014, with around 600 million of them classified as obese. The Global Burden of Disease study for the United States identified high body mass index (BMI) and physical inactivity as possibly preventable risk factors contributing to the increase in disease burden, resulting in the loss of healthy years [27]. The concept of healthy years refers to the projected lifespan of an individual at a specific age, during which they can anticipate being free from any form of disability or activity constraint. Despite an increase in the levels of adequate physical activity among both males and females, only nine countries in the United States observed a drop in obesity rates between 2001 and 2009. However, it is important to note that these results were statistically insignificant when compared to the increase in obesity rates observed in the remaining countries . The systematic analysis conducted by Mehmood and Papandreou [27] aimed to examine the prevalence of overweight and obesity in children and adults on a global, regional, and national scale from 1980 to 2013. The public health sector must prioritize the investigation and resolution of socio-economic consequences associated with the maintenance of Vitamin D levels. Possible mechanisms that account for the insufficiency of this fat-soluble vitamin in individuals with an excess of adipocytes include altered metabolism, sequestration in adipose tissue, altered dietary intake, and behavior resulting in decreased cutaneous synthesis, synthetic capacity, and intestinal absorption [27]. The phenomenon of autophagy down-regulation in hepatocyte lipid droplets in the liver, which is linked to obesity, results in the buildup of triglycerides, endoplasmic reticulum stress, and insulin resistance [27]. To summarize, the presence of visceral fat in contrast to subcutaneous fat can potentially lead to metabolic dysfunctions due to the release of inflammatory adipokines, including interleukin, tumor necrosis factor-α, macrophage chemoattractant protein-1, and resistin. These adipokines can induce insulin resistance, diabetes, and disturbances in Vitamin D metabolism [27].

The expression of the Vitamin D receptor (VDR) is notably elevated in adipose tissues and exhibits sensitivity to the fat-soluble compound, 1,25(OH)2D [28]. There exists a substantial and inverse correlation between elevated body fat and increased body mass index (BMI) with blood 25-hydroxyvitamin D (25(OH)D) levels. The human body has been recognized to utilize body fat as a reservoir for the storage of vitamin D. Obesity is a contributing factor to the development of vitamin D insufficiency, which in turn has been associated with weight increase [28]. Due to the lipid solubility of vitamin D metabolites, any surplus of circulating 25(OH)D is drawn towards adipose tissue. Hence, individuals who have surplus body fat should consume oral vitamin D supplements in greater quantities or be exposed to the sun for extended periods (*i.e.*, body mass and adiposity should be considered when determining the vitamin D dietary needs of the obese) [28].

Diabetes

This section will provide a summary of the impact of vitamin D on those with prediabetes, diabetes, and those without diabetes.

Diabetes encompasses not just impaired glucose regulation but also has an inflammatory component. The beneficial impacts of vitamin D on islet-cell functions, insulin release, and insulin resistance reduction can be attributed to its anti-inflammatory properties [28]. The insufficiency of vitamin D not only increases the susceptibility of persons to acquire type 1 Diabetes (T1D) and T2D, but it also results in suboptimal reactions to treatment [28]. Vitamin D is additionally involved in insulin signaling, hence influencing the susceptibility to diabetes. A study conducted in Norway, based on population data, revealed a significant negative correlation between increased body mass index (BMI) and lowered levels of vitamin D. Furthermore, there was an observed inverse correlation between serum 25(OH)D levels and both the average blood sugar concentrations and the degree of insulin resistance. The identification of vitamin D receptors within the pancreatic β-cells provides additional evidence to support the notion that vitamin D plays a role in the regulation of insulin production and secretion. Fig. (**3**) depicts the prevailing pathways that result in the deterioration of β-cells and the subsequent onset of diabetes. Additionally, it presents the potential impact of vitamin D in mitigating these processes, hence implying the involvement of vitamin D in the development of IR, as well as the indirect effects on glucotoxicity and lipotoxicity. According to Wimalawansa [28], a deficit in vitamin D results in a detrimental cycle characterized by the exacerbation of IR, impairment of β-cell function, and the subsequent onset of diabetes.

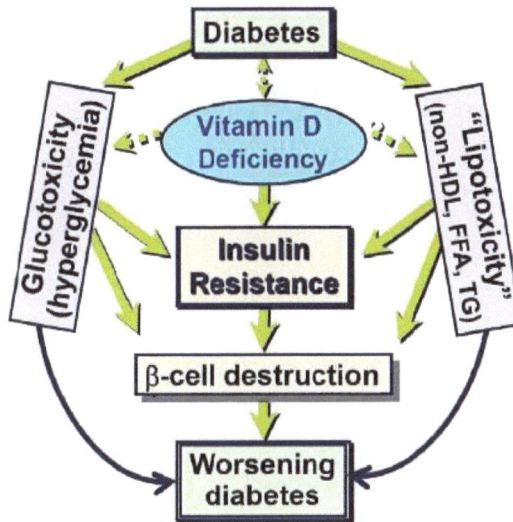

Fig. (3). Role of vitamin D deficiency and IR in the development of diabetes. Adapted with permission [28].

Research studies have provided evidence to support the notion that the utilization of Vitamin D supplements can yield beneficial effects on insulin resistance. This is achieved by the enhancement of glucose biomarkers in individuals, irrespective of whether they have been diagnosed with diabetes or not. Insulin resistance frequently contributes to the advancement of T2D. The pathophysiology of T2D is characterized by a decrease in the bulk of β-cells and a decline in β-cell activity [29]. Dysfunction of β-cells can lead to impaired or insufficient insulin secretion, hence compromising glucose homeostasis. Previous research has demonstrated that vitamin D can stimulate pancreatic β-cells, hence facilitating the maintenance of insulin secretion [29]. According to Sarkar [29], the administration of vitamin D has been found to enhance the process of autophagy while concurrently decreasing the likelihood of apoptosis in pancreatic β-cells, as depicted in Fig. (**4**). In contrast to T2D, the onset of T1D is attributed to the destruction of pancreatic β-cells driven by autoimmune. According to Sarkar [29], the administration of vitamin D supplementation resulted in the restoration of pancreatic β-cell functioning in a mouse model of T1D.

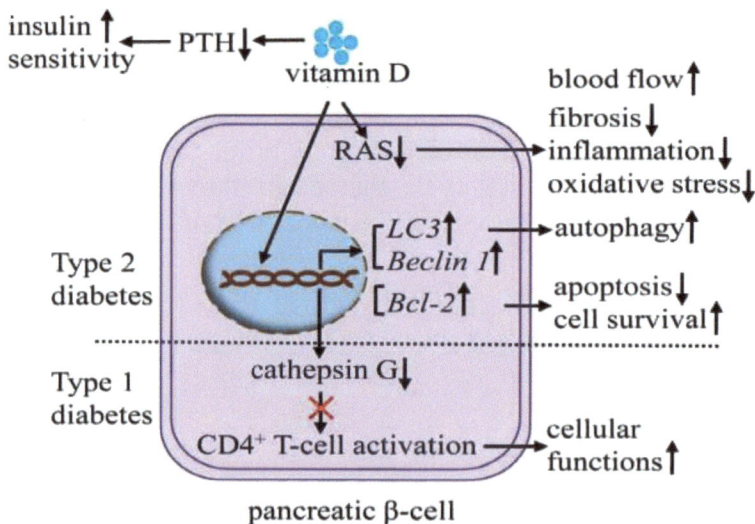

Fig. (4). Role of vitamin D in regulating molecular pathways linked to diabetes. Adapted with permission [29].

Rafiq and Jeppesen [30] conducted a systematic review and meta-analysis involving a total of 40 studies, encompassing participants both with and without diabetes. The findings revealed a significant negative association between vitamin D levels and IR in both non-diabetic ($p = 0.000$) and diabetic populations ($p = 0.001$), with a stronger correlation observed in individuals with diabetes. The study found a significant negative correlation between vitamin D levels and IR, regardless of the participant's age and gender. According to the meta-analysis, it was shown that insufficient levels of vitamin D may contribute to elevated IR in individuals with and without diabetes. Furthermore, the findings obtained from the subgroup analysis, which was conducted based on BMI, revealed a significant negative association between vitamin D levels and IR as BMI increased among the non-diabetic participants. According to the study conducted by Rafiq and Jeppesen [30], there exists an inverse relationship between IR and the level of vitamin D in both individuals with diabetes and those without diabetes.

The impact of vitamin D supplementation in individuals with prediabetes has been a topic of debate and disagreement. The findings of a systematic review examining the impact of vitamin D supplementation on the reduction of IR indicate that, among the eight trials analyzed, only one trial demonstrated a potential improvement in insulin resistance or a decrease in the risk of developing T2D in individuals with prediabetes. A single study demonstrated enhancements in FBG and HOMA-IR, as reported by Pieńkowska *et al.* [31]. It is worth noting that there is a significant occurrence of low levels of vitamin D among individuals with diabetes. According to a cross-sectional study conducted by Vijay *et al.* [32], it was observed that out of a total of 116 patients diagnosed with diabetes, 86 individuals were found to exhibit a deficiency in vitamin D.

Mirhosseini *et al.* [33] conducted a meta-analysis to examine the impact of vitamin D supplementation on the enhancement of glycemic control and reduction of IR in individuals diagnosed with T2D. A total of 24 clinical trials, involving a total of 1528 patients diagnosed with T2D, were included. The analysis included data from 23 studies which consisted of 1477 diabetic patients, showing that vitamin D supplementation significantly decreased HbA1c levels (p= <0.001). A pooled analysis of 21 studies, which involved 1386 patients used FBG as an outcome measure. The results showed a significant decrease in FBG levels after the supplementation of vitamin D, as indicated by a p-value of 0.003. A total of twelve studies were employed to assess the collective impact of vitamin D supplementation on IR, as measured by the HOMA-IR. Among the 12 studies examined, it was seen that 7 of them demonstrated a statistically significant decline in IR after the administration of vitamin D supplements, as compared to the placebo group. Conversely, the remaining 5 studies did not yield such a reduction. The study concluded that administering a minimum dose of 100mg/day (4000I IU/day) of vitamin D could lead to a significant decrease in FPG, HbA1c, and HOMA-IR index. These findings indicate that administering vitamin D supplements may assist in regulating blood sugar levels and enhancing the body's responsiveness to insulin in individuals with T2D [33].

Metabolic Syndrome (MS)

Metabolic syndrome, often known as MS, is a collection of metabolic abnormalities that encompass abdominal obesity, heightened FBG levels, elevated blood pressure (BP), increased triglyceride levels, and reduced high-density lipoprotein cholesterol (HDL-C) levels. MS has been found to exhibit a robust correlation with elevated rates of morbidity, mortality, and healthcare expenditures [34]. The global prevalence of MS varies between 10% and 84%, depending on factors such as the definition employed, the sex and race of the individuals, and the geographical distribution of the population being examined [35]. The main strategy for managing this condition is altering the underlying environmental risk factors, such as excess body weight, a sedentary lifestyle, a diet that promotes atherosclerosis, smoking, and alcohol intake [36].

Vitamin D is classified as a fat-soluble prohormone and has historically been linked to the regulation of bone mineral metabolism [36]. Over time, there have been proposed additional non-skeletal functions of vitamin D. In recent times, there has been an increasing body of research that establishes a connection between insufficient levels of vitamin D and MS as well as its components. The proposed correlation between these two phenomena was posited based on the significant overlap in risk factors, including insufficient physical activity and limited exposure to sunlight [36]. Research has indicated that insufficient amounts of vitamin D result in reduced intracellular calcium concentrations, impeding the release of insulin by cells and hence diminishing glucose tolerance. In addition, it should be noted that vitamin D has been found to enhance the quantity of insulin receptors, a critical factor in promoting insulin sensitivity and regulating glucose metabolism. Moreover, vitamin D possesses hormonal, anti-inflammatory, anti-fibrotic and anti-apoptotic properties, suggesting its potential in the prevention of MS [36].

Theik *et al.* [37] conducted a systematic review that examined the relationship between vitamin D and various components of MS. The analysis examined observational data that showed a substantial association between vitamin D levels and MS, including obesity, dyslipidemia, blood pressure, and glucose metabolism. Furthermore, empirical evidence suggests that vitamin D supplementation has a positive effect on these markers. A recent systematic review and meta-analysis conducted by Lee and Kim [38] demonstrated that an elevation of 10 ng/mL in vitamin D concentration was associated with a reduction of 20% and 15% in the likelihood of developing MS in cross-sectional and cohort studies, respectively.

Conversely, a recent investigation by Abboud *et al.* [36] found no significant correlation between serum vitamin D levels and MS while controlling for age, gender, and other lifestyle factors like physical activity, sleep patterns, stress levels, food addiction, and smoking habits. Individuals diagnosed with MS had marginally elevated levels of serum vitamin D when compared to those without MS. Nevertheless, it is important to note that this observed correlation did not reach statistical significance. The existing body of information pertaining to the relationship between vitamin D and MS displays a lack of consistency. Several studies have demonstrated a negative correlation between the variables under investigation [39], but other investigations have not documented a similar relationship [40].

Moreover, there remains ambiguity over the specific constituents of MS that may be implicated in this correlation, as certain investigations propose a link with obesity, while others propose a link with glucose homeostasis. Further research is necessary to establish a causal link between vitamin D and MS as well as metabolic disorders, thus warranting future interventional investigations. In light of the extensive occurrence of vitamin D insufficiency, it is recommended that immediate measures be implemented on a national scale to effectively tackle the issue and mitigate potential repercussions [36].

Polycystic Ovary Syndrome (PCOS)

PCOS is the most prevalent endocrine condition among women in their reproductive years. PCOS has a significant impact on a substantial proportion of women, with a prevalence that might potentially surpass 10-15%, contingent upon the specific diagnostic criteria employed and the populations investigated in various geographic regions [41]. PCOS is a medical condition that affects multiple systems in the body. It is defined by infrequent or absent ovulation, leading to irregular or absent menstrual periods, as well as the development of excessive quantities of male hormones (hyperandrogenism). These hormonal imbalances are caused by elevated levels of luteinizing hormone (LH) in the bloodstream and an altered ratio of LH to follicle stimulating hormone (FSH) [42]. Polycystic ovarian morphology (PCOM) is a term used to describe the morphological presentation of the ovaries, characterized by the presence of many cysts. Polycystic ovary syndrome (PCOS) has been found to be correlated with hyperinsulinemia, poor glucose tolerance, and occasionally T2D [42]. Additional factors, including IR, dyslipidemia, and systemic inflammation, contribute to the constellation of signs and symptoms observed in patients with PCOS and increase their susceptibility to cardiovascular disease compared to those without PCOS [43]. The occurrence of impaired insulin sensitivity is likely to result in a compensatory hyperinsulinemia, which plays a role in the development of hyperandrogenism by chronically stimulating the cells of the ovarian theca. Research findings have indicated a connection between the development of IR and a lack of vitamin D, so implicating insufficient levels of VD as a contributing factor to the occurrence of metabolic syndrome in women with PCOS [42]. The expression of the vitamin D receptor (VDR) is nearly ubiquitous, exerting regulatory control over approximately 3% of the human genome, including genes involved in glucose metabolism [44]. This implies the relationship and association between vitamin D insufficiency and symptoms of PCOS such as T2D, IR, and cardiovascular illnesses. Morgante *et al.* [42] conducted a meta-analysis to examine the association between vitamin D receptor polymorphisms and PCOS, as well as to discover potential susceptibility markers. The utilization of metformin in individuals with PCOS is considered a significant advancement in the treatment of this patient population [45]. According to Morgante *et al.* [42], the administration of natural compounds, such as vitamin D, could potentially alleviate symptoms associated with PCOS.

It is noteworthy that recent research has demonstrated a potential exacerbation of PCOS symptoms due to low levels of vitamin D. In fact, a negative relationship has been observed between blood VD levels and the metabolic and hormonal imbalances associated with PCOS, as reported by Grzesiak [46]. Limited research has been conducted on the correlation between vitamin D insufficiency and PCOS characteristics. In their study, Davis *et al.* [47] analyzed women diagnosed with PCOS. These women were categorized into three different diagnostic phenotypes based on the Rotterdam criteria. The study population is comprised of three distinct groups: (i) women with ovulatory dysfunction and polycystic ovaries comprise group 1; (ii) women with androgen excess and ovulatory dysfunction comprise group 2; and (iii) women with ovulatory dysfunction attributable to both polycystic ovaries and androgen excess collectively comprise group 3. The study conducted by Davis *et al.* [47] indicates that there is a type of PCOS that also exhibits excessive levels of androgens. Maktabi and colleagues conducted a randomized controlled experiment to investigate the effects of a placebo in women with vitamin D deficiency (serum concentrations less than 20 ng/mL), who exhibited phenotypic B-PCOS based on the Rotterdam criteria [48]. According to Maktabi *et al.* [48], the administration of VD supplementation throughout a 12-week intervention resulted in a significant reduction in FBG, insulin, and HOMA-IR index. Additionally, it was shown that quantitative insulin sensitivity enhanced as a result of the intervention. Fig. (**5**) depicts the key mechanisms that are vital in the direct and indirect impact of vitamin D on the development of IR and MS in PCOS, hormonal imbalance, and infertility [42].

In a recent study, Zhang *et al.* [49] performed a meta-analysis of randomized controlled trials (RCTs) to assess the impact of vitamin D supplementation on individuals diagnosed with PCOS. The objective of this research was to contribute trustworthy information to inform the therapeutic management of PCOS. A total of thirteen RCTs involving a sample size of 840 patients diagnosed with PCOS were incorporated into the analysis. The findings of meta-analytic studies have demonstrated a substantial association between vitamin D supplementation and an increase in serum vitamin D levels. Additionally, this supplementation has been shown to lead to a reduction in serum levels of lipid, glycemic and inflammatory markers. In addition, it has been noted that vitamin D has the ability to impede the production of peroxisome proliferator-activated receptor gamma (PPAR-γ) and hinder the transformation of preadipocytes into adipocytes. Consequently, this mechanism serves to counteract adipogenesis and diminish insulin resistance in peripheral tissues [49]. Hence, it may be inferred that the administration of vitamin D has the potential to enhance the lipid profile of individuals with PCOS who are obese, consequently leading to a reduction in BMI and an overall improvement in the obesity condition of these patients. According to Zhang *et al.* [49], it has been observed that following therapy with a vitamin D3 analog, there is an increase in insulin secretion during the initial phase, along with notable improvements in lipid profiles.

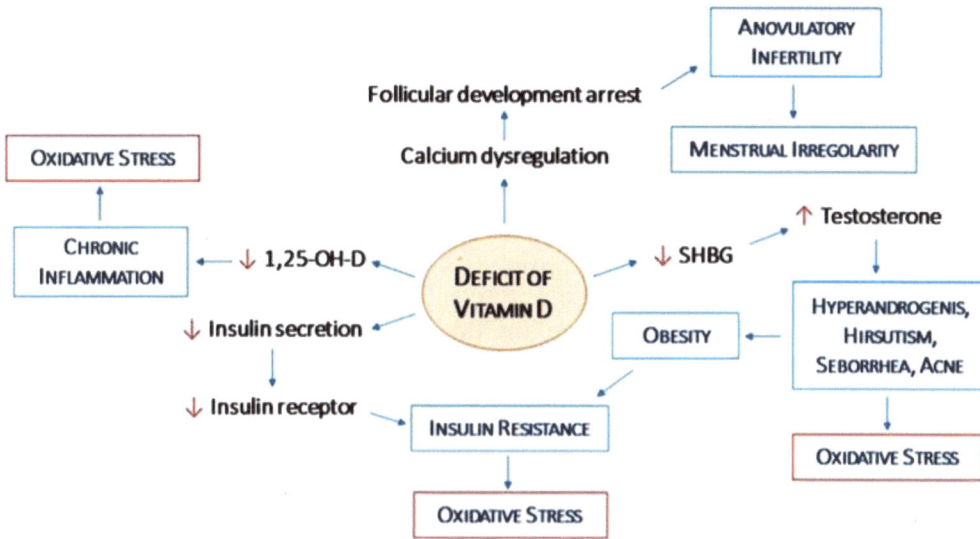

Fig. (5). Correlation between vitamin D deficiency and the development of IR, MS, hormonal imbalance, and infertility in PCOS. Adapted with permission [42].

Additionally, in a recent study conducted by Cochrane *et al.* [50], a systematic review and meta-analysis were performed on PCOS. The findings of this study indicated that women with PCOS exhibit a positive response to vitamin D supplementation. However, it was seen that the potential benefits derived from administering doses over 3000 IU per day were small. Additional evidence is necessary to ascertain the dose-response relationship at dosages beyond 5000 IU/day, as well as to evaluate if larger intakes offer any significant clinical benefits in this particular population.

Non-alcoholic Fatty Liver Disease (NAFLD)

Nonalcoholic fatty liver disease (NAFLD) is a prevalent condition described by the accumulation of fat deposits, without the presence of excess alcohol intake or other well-documented etiologies of hepatic injury [51]. The condition can be categorized into two primary forms: the non-progressive form, referred to as NAFLD, which has a low likelihood of progressing to cirrhosis, and the progressive form, known as nonalcoholic steatohepatitis (NASH), which is associated with the development of cirrhosis and hepatocellular carcinoma [51]. NAFLD, which is strongly associated with obesity and IR, represents a widely recognized chronic liver disease that affects individuals across many age groups [52]. There exists substantial evidence indicating a strong association between the excessive intake of diets high in fat and sugar-sweetened beverages and the development and progression NAFLD. Moreover, the ingestion of an excessive amount of carbohydrates and fats has been found to elevate blood sugar levels and free fatty acid concentrations, leading to an excessive accumulation of neutral lipids in the liver [51].

The overconsumption of fructose has been discovered to worsen the severity of NAFLD because it promotes IR, the production of fat (lipogenesis), and the development of inflammation and oxidative stress [53]. The therapy and control of NAFLD are of great significance due to its connection with irregular hepatic enzymes, cirrhosis, and liver transplantation [51]. Multiple lines of evidence indicate that vitamin D has the ability to regulate liver inflammation and enhance the liver's sensitivity to insulin through its interaction with the particular receptor in the liver [54]. The study conducted by Liu *et al.* [55] provides evidence supporting the notion that an active form of vitamin D has the potential to mitigate oxidative stress, suppress the production of inflammatory markers, and alleviate hepatic fibrosis in NAFLD induced by a high-fat diet. According to Liu *et al.* [55], the modulation of lipid metabolism and/or inhibition of cell senescence may contribute to the alleviation of fatty liver disease in a NAFLD rat model. Furthermore, the consumption of vitamin D has the potential to mitigate the severity of NAFLD as well as its associated risk factors such as dyslipidemia and obesity, as suggested by Sangouni *et al.* [56].

Chen *et al.* [57] recently performed a systematic review and meta-analysis encompassing eight randomized controlled trials (RCTs) involving a total of 657 patients. The objective of the study was to assess the impact of vitamin D supplementation on individuals diagnosed with NAFLD. The study's results indicated a considerable increase in 25(OH)D levels as a result of Vitamin D supplementation. Additionally, the study found a significant impact of vitamin D supplementation on the insulin resistance index. A study conducted by Mehmood and Papandreou [27] in adult individuals revealed a robust association between vitamin D and NAFLD. The study conducted by the authors used a sample size of 1081 adults. Their findings indicated a strong correlation between low levels of vitamin D and NAFLD in individuals with diabetes or IR. This association was observed to be irrespective of the presence of visceral obesity.

Hence, it is suggested that the administration of vitamin D supplements may offer potential benefits in mitigating the occurrence of NAFLD through the modulation of certain serum markers and specific molecules associated with inflammatory and anti-inflammatory processes, as well as the mRNA expression levels of regulatory molecules involved in the regulation of lipolysis, lipogenesis, and insulin signalling [51].

Diabetic Kidney Disease (DKD)

Diabetic kidney disease (DKD) is a significant causative factor in the progression to end-stage renal disease on a global level. Multiple studies have been guided to substantiate the role of vitamin D as a kidney-protective drug, demonstrating its capacity to delay the onset of DKD. The physiological impacts of vitamin D are facilitated through its interaction with a receptor that is widely distributed among several organs inside the human body, including the kidneys. It is worth mentioning that this receptor is present in both the proximal and distal tubular epithelial cells. The findings indicate that the kidneys have a pivotal function in the regulation of vitamin D metabolism by exerting control over calcium and phosphate reabsorption, as well as modulating the synthesis of the biologically active form of vitamin D [58].

Huang *et al.* [59] conducted a review to present a comprehensive summary of recent scientific investigations about the relationship between vitamin D and its effects on DKD. Numerous animal and clinical investigations have shown evidence supporting a negative correlation between reduced levels of vitamin D and the likelihood of developing DKD. This review article presents an analysis of the main outcomes derived from 14 studies completed from 2012 to 2021, with a specific emphasis on the application of vitamin D therapy in individuals diagnosed with DKD. The aforementioned investigations encompass a total of ten RCTs, two prospective observational studies, and two cross-sectional studies.

The randomized controlled studies utilized varying population inclusion criteria, specifically based on eGFR ranges. In addition, it should be noted that the randomized controlled trials (RCTs) discussed in the study did not employ a standardized dosage of vitamin D across the various research populations. After analyzing a total of 10 randomized controlled trials (RCTs), it was concluded that in five of these trials, there were no statistically significant disparities observed in the estimated glomerular filtration rate (eGFR) between the groups receiving vitamin D therapy and those receiving a placebo. This result was derived from the fact that the p-values associated with all of these investigations exceeded the threshold of 0.05. The empirical evidence substantiating this discovery encompasses the investigations carried out by Krairittichai *et al.* [60], Barzegari *et al.* [61], Ahmadi *et al.* [62], Tiryaki *et al.* [63], and Thethi *et al.* [64]. Nevertheless, three studies have documented statistically significant alterations in the eGFR when comparing the treatment group to the placebo group subsequent to the administration of vitamin D. This is supported by the observation that all reported p-values in the aforementioned investigations were below the threshold of 0.05 [60, 62, 63]. The evaluation of glomerular filtration rate (GFR) subsequent to the therapy was not carried out in two investigations, specifically Munisamy *et al.* [65] and Liyanage *et al.* [66].

In a prospective observational study conducted by Mao *et al.* [67], the aim was to assess the effectiveness of providing oral vitamin D at a daily dose of 0.25 µg for a duration of 6 months in a cohort of 24 persons diagnosed with T1D and exhibiting elevated levels of microalbuminuria. The findings of the study indicated a statistically significant reduction in urine albumin excretion, with levels decreasing from 127.05 to 104.81 µg/mg (p < 0.05). Nevertheless, the study did not see any substantial enhancement in glucose metabolism, potentially because to an inadequate sample size. In a prospective observational study conducted by Kim *et al.* [68], the primary aim was to assess the effectiveness of providing oral vitamin D3 at a dosage of 40,000 IU per week for a length of 8 weeks on estimated glomerular filtration rate (eGFR) at 2 and 4 months. The study findings indicated that there were no statistically significant disparities in the eGFR between the treatment group after 2 months (42 to 41 mL/min/1.73 m2, p > 0.05) and after 4 months (42 to 40 mL/min/1.73 m2, p > 0.05).

Bonakdaran *et al.* [69] utilized a cross-sectional research design to examine the effects of vitamin D therapy on multiple health indicators in a cohort of 119 individuals diagnosed with T2D and exhibiting elevated levels of albuminuria. The study findings indicated that the administration of vitamin D yielded significant improvements in glycosylated hemoglobin (p = 0.014), reduction of diastolic blood pressure (p = 0.004), total cholesterol levels (p = 0.019), low-density lipoprotein levels (p = 0.04), and high-density lipoprotein levels (p = 0.001). In a cross-sectional study conducted by Huang *et al.* [70], the objective was to assess the effects of oral vitamin D3 supplementation, administered at a daily dosage of 800 IU over a period of 6 months, on the eGFR in people diagnosed with T2D and exhibiting a urine albumin-to-creatinine ratio (UACR) over 30 mg/g. The study findings revealed that there was no statistically significant disparity in eGFR levels before and after the administration of vitamin D3 supplementation in the treatment group (97.39 to 120.36 mg/g, p = 0.239).

Diabetic Peripheral Neuropathy (DPN)

Diabetic peripheral neuropathy (DPN) is a condition characterized by the long-term nerve damage that occurs as a result of diabetes mellitus. The simultaneous presence of metabolic factors, such as IR, hypertension, and obesity, may be noticed in association with it. In the research conducted by Sharma *et al.* [71], it was observed that a prevalent indicator of DPN is the manifestation of a diabetic foot ulcer. The disease being examined is a clinical state characterized by the co-occurrence of neuropathy and ischaemia in the lower extremities of individuals diagnosed with diabetes. Individuals with diabetes have significant challenges in terms of the prevalence of limb amputation, mortality rates, disability, economic implications, and diminished quality of life. In addition, individuals may also be prone to developing a vitamin D deficit. Furthermore, a study conducted by Kinesya *et al.* [72] has demonstrated the effects of vitamin D on immunological response, insulin production, and insulin sensitivity.

The study undertaken by Iqhrammullah *et al.* [73] involved a thorough examination to explore the correlation between serum vitamin D levels and the incidence of diabetic foot ulcers (DFU). The primary objective of the researchers was to acquire a deeper understanding of the fundamental pathogenic mechanism implicated in this association. A thorough investigation was conducted across a total of 12 databases in order to gather relevant literature that had been published up until the stipulated date of March 10, 2023. The systematic review conducted a comprehensive analysis of twenty-one studies, which collectively involved a total of 9,570 participants. A total of 18 papers were considered appropriate for inclusion in the meta-analysis. The study utilized a research style that incorporated both retrospective and prospective observational studies. The analysis was constrained to research that were published solely in either the English or Indonesian language. The study implemented exclusion criteria to determine eligibility for participation. These criteria included the exclusion of pregnant and lactating women, as well as persons with a past history of regular consumption of vitamin D, calcium supplements, or immune suppressants prior to the initiation of the research.

Seven studies have provided evidence indicating a higher occurrence of individuals with insufficient glycemic control in the cohort of patients with DFUs compared to the cohort without DFUs [74 - 79]. Moreover, a cross-sectional study conducted by Tiwari *et al.* [80] revealed that people exhibiting severe hypovitaminosis D (less than 25 nmol/L) had a significantly greater prevalence of

DFU in comparison to both the DFU group and the diabetic control group (48.2% *versus* 20.5%, respectively). The group of individuals with DFU exhibited a statistically significant reduction in vitamin D levels as compared to the group of individuals without DFU. The meta-analysis included a majority of cross-sectional studies that presented data supporting the notion of reduced serum vitamin D levels in individuals with DFU, with the exception of the study conducted by Afarideh *et al.* [79]. Therefore, a significant association has been identified between insufficient levels of vitamin D and an increased prevalence of DFU, as evidenced by a comprehensive review of many studies. In addition, Lin *et al.* [81] conducted a meta-analysis that incorporated a comprehensive set of 12 investigations. The research conducted in this study consisted of four case-control studies, three prospective cohort studies, three cross-sectional studies, and two retrospective investigations. The aforementioned publications were published between the years 2013 and 2022. The entire study population consisted of 7586 individuals who had been diagnosed with diabetes mellitus. Among the entire sample, a subgroup consisting of 1565 patients displayed DFU wounds, but the remaining 6021 people did not manifest any ulcerated wounds. The findings suggest a significant decline in vitamin D levels in individuals with diabetes who have diabetic foot ulcers (DFU) ($p < .004$). Furthermore, it has been noted that these individuals demonstrate a higher frequency of vitamin D insufficiency, which is specifically defined as a level below 50 nmoL/L ($p < .001$), as well as a greater prevalence of severe vitamin D deficiency ($p < .001$).

In contrast, Iqhrammullah *et al.* [73] conducted a review of five additional studies that sought to determine the proportion of patients with HbA1c levels exceeding 8%, which is indicative of insufficient glycemic control. These studies aimed to establish a comparable distribution of such patients between the group with DFU and the control group without DFU [80, 82 - 84]. Furthermore, the study cited above provided evidence that the statistical significance of a regression model utilizing the HbA1c level as the independent variable was restricted. This suggests that the extent of glycation control did not have a significant effect on the blood vitamin D level. Likewise, it was shown that the variety within the collective study cohort remained unaltered in relation to nutritional status. However, it was shown that the apparent heterogeneity in the study was impacted by additional factors, such as age and geography. In conclusion, the probability of DFU being impacted by a deficiency in vitamin D is diminished, considering its tendency to add to the exacerbation of IR. However, it is crucial to recognize that further research is necessary in order to fully understand the relationship between vitamin D and IR in the setting of DFU.

CONCLUSION AND RECOMMENDATIONS

In summary, the current body of research indicates that Vitamin D functions as an immunomodulator of significant importance, influencing critical human conditions such as insulin resistance and glucose homeostasis, in addition to regulating mineral and bone metabolism. A large body of evidence indicates that vitamin D plays a significant role in the development of IR, involving various gene variations connected to vitamin D and metabolic and immunological pathways associated with vitamin D. Supplementing with vitamin D may help effectively manage and improve IR. Various research methodologies have produced both positive and negative outcomes about the association between vitamin D and IR. Additional investigation is advised to elucidate the relationship between vitamin D and insulin function, as well as to ascertain potential disparities in this connection among distinct age groups, genders, and disorders.

REFERENCES

[1]   Aedh AI, Alshahrani MS, Huneif MA, Pryme IF, Oruch R. A glimpse into milestones of insulin resistance and an updated review of its management. Nutrients 2023; 15(4): 921.
        [http://dx.doi.org/10.3390/nu15040921] [PMID: 36839279]

[2]   Freeman AM, Acevedo LA, Pennings N. Insulin Resistance 2024.

[3]   Fahed M, Abou Jaoudeh MG, Merhi S, *et al.* Evaluation of risk factors for insulin resistance: a cross sectional study among employees at a private university in Lebanon. BMC Endocr Disord 2020; 20(1): 85.
        [http://dx.doi.org/10.1186/s12902-020-00558-9] [PMID: 32522257]

[4]   Gołacki J, Matuszek M, Matyjaszek-Matuszek B. Link between insulin resistance and obesity—from diagnosis to treatment. Diagnostics (Basel) 2022; 12(7): 1681.
        [http://dx.doi.org/10.3390/diagnostics12071681] [PMID: 35885586]

[5]   Trimarco V, Manzi MV, Mancusi C, *et al.* Insulin resistance and vitamin D deficiency: A link beyond the appearances. Front Cardiovasc Med 2022; 9: 859793.
        [http://dx.doi.org/10.3389/fcvm.2022.859793] [PMID: 35369303]

[6]   Landau Z, Raz I, Wainstein J, Bar-Dayan Y, Cahn A. The role of insulin pump therapy for type 2 diabetes mellitus. Diabetes Metab Res Rev 2017; 33(1): e2822.
        [http://dx.doi.org/10.1002/dmrr.2822] [PMID: 27189155]

[7]   Lemieux P, Weisnagel SJ, Caron AZ, *et al.* Effects of 6-month vitamin D supplementation on insulin sensitivity and secretion: a randomised, placebo-controlled trial. Eur J Endocrinol 2019; 181(3): 287-99.
        [http://dx.doi.org/10.1530/EJE-19-0156] [PMID: 31344685]

[8]   Contreras-Bolívar V, García-Fontana B, García-Fontana C, Muñoz-Torres M. Mechanisms involved in the relationship between vitamin D and insulin resistance: Impact on clinical practice. Nutrients 2021; 13(10): 3491.
        [http://dx.doi.org/10.3390/nu13103491] [PMID: 34684492]

[9]   Sharafi SM, Yazdi M, Goodarzi-Khoigani M, Kelishadi R. Effect of vitamin D supplementation on serum 25-hydroxyvitamin D and homeostatic model of insulin resistance levels in healthy pregnancy: A systematic review and meta-analysis. Iran J Med Sci 2023; 48(1): 4-12.
        [PMID: 36688198]

[10] Kim KS, Park SW, Cho YW, Kim SK, Vitamin D. Vitamin D deficiency at mid-pregnancy is associated with a higher risk of postpartum glucose intolerance in women with gestational diabetes mellitus. Endocrinol Metab (Seoul) 2020; 35(1): 97-105.
[http://dx.doi.org/10.3803/EnM.2020.35.1.97] [PMID: 32207269]

[11] Rodrigues CZ, Cardoso MA, Maruyama JM, Neves PAR, Qi L, Lourenço BH. Vitamin D insufficiency, excessive weight gain, and insulin resistance during pregnancy. Nutr Metab Cardiovasc Dis 2022; 32(9): 2121-8.
[http://dx.doi.org/10.1016/j.numecd.2022.05.009] [PMID: 35843794]

[12] Hofman-Hutna J, Hutny M, Matusik E, Olszanecka-Glinianowicz M, Matusik P, Vitamin D. Vitamin D deficiency in obese children is associated with some metabolic syndrome components, but not with metabolic syndrome itself. Metabolites 2023; 13(8): 914.
[http://dx.doi.org/10.3390/metabo13080914] [PMID: 37623858]

[13] Corsello A, Macchi M, D'Oria V, *et al.* Effects of vitamin D supplementation in obese and overweight children and adolescents: A systematic review and meta-analysis. Pharmacol Res 2023; 192: 106793.
[http://dx.doi.org/10.1016/j.phrs.2023.106793] [PMID: 37178775]

[14] Belenchia AM, Tosh AK, Hillman LS, Peterson CA. Correcting vitamin D insufficiency improves insulin sensitivity in obese adolescents: a randomized controlled trial. Am J Clin Nutr 2013; 97(4): 774-81.
[http://dx.doi.org/10.3945/ajcn.112.050013] [PMID: 23407306]

[15] Kelishadi R, Salek S, Salek M, Hashemipour M, Movahedian M. Effects of vitamin D supplementation on insulin resistance and cardiometabolic risk factors in children with metabolic syndrome: a triple-masked controlled trial. J Pediatr (Rio J) 2014; 90(1): 28-34.
[http://dx.doi.org/10.1016/j.jped.2013.06.006] [PMID: 24140383]

[16] Rajakumar K, Moore CG, Khalid AT, *et al.* Effect of vitamin D3 supplementation on vascular and metabolic health of vitamin D–deficient overweight and obese children: a randomized clinical trial. Am J Clin Nutr 2020; 111(4): 757-68.
[http://dx.doi.org/10.1093/ajcn/nqz340] [PMID: 31950134]

[17] Rostampour N, Asadpour N, Moradi M, Hashemi-Dehkordi E, Kheiri S. Effect of Vitamin D on insulin resistance in overweight and obese children and adolescents with vitamin D deficiency. Acta Med Iran 2020.
[http://dx.doi.org/10.18502/acta.v58i2.3711]

[18] Sethuraman U, Zidan MA, Hanks L, Bagheri M, Ashraf A. Impact of vitamin D treatment on 25 hydroxy vitamin D levels and insulin homeostasis in obese African American adolescents in a randomized trial. J Clin Transl Endocrinol 2018; 12: 13-9.
[http://dx.doi.org/10.1016/j.jcte.2018.03.002] [PMID: 29892562]

[19] Vinet A, Morrissey C, Perez-Martin A, *et al.* Effect of vitamin D supplementation on microvascular reactivity in obese adolescents: A randomized controlled trial. Nutr Metab Cardiovasc Dis 2021; 31(8): 2474-83.
[http://dx.doi.org/10.1016/j.numecd.2021.04.025] [PMID: 34090775]

[20] De Cosmi V, Mazzocchi A, D'Oria V, *et al.* Effect of vitamin D and docosahexaenoic acid co-supplementation on vitamin d status, body composition, and metabolic markers in obese children: A Randomized, Double Blind, Controlled Study. Nutrients 2022; 14(7): 1397.
[http://dx.doi.org/10.3390/nu14071397] [PMID: 35406010]

[21] Javed A, Vella A, Balagopal PB, *et al.* Cholecalciferol supplementation does not influence β-cell function and insulin action in obese adolescents: a prospective double-blind randomized trial. J Nutr 2015; 145(2): 284-90.
[http://dx.doi.org/10.3945/jn.114.202010] [PMID: 25644349]

[22] Javed A, Kullo IJ, Balagopal PB, Kumar S. Effect of vitamin D_3 treatment on endothelial function in obese adolescents. Pediatr Obes 2016; 11(4): 279-84.

[http://dx.doi.org/10.1111/ijpo.12059] [PMID: 26273791]

[23]   Magge SN, Prasad D, Zemel BS, Kelly A. Vitamin D3 supplementation in obese, African-American, vitamin D deficient adolescents. J Clin Transl Endocrinol 2018; 12: 1-7.
[http://dx.doi.org/10.1016/j.jcte.2018.03.001] [PMID: 29892560]

[24]   Nader NS, Aguirre Castaneda R, Wallace J, Singh R, Weaver A, Kumar S. Effect of vitamin D3 supplementation on serum 25(OH)D, lipids and markers of insulin resistance in obese adolescents: a prospective, randomized, placebo-controlled pilot trial. Horm Res Paediatr 2014; 82(2): 107-12.
[http://dx.doi.org/10.1159/000362449] [PMID: 25034315]

[25]   Samaranayake DBDL, Adikaram SGS, Atapattu N, *et al.* Vitamin D supplementation in obese Sri Lankan children: a randomized controlled trial. BMC Pediatr 2020; 20(1): 426.
[http://dx.doi.org/10.1186/s12887-020-02329-w] [PMID: 32891139]

[26]   Khadgawat R, Varshney S, Gahlot M, *et al.* Effect of high-dose vitamin D supplementation on beta cell function in obese Asian-Indian children and adolescents: A randomized, double blind, active controlled study. Indian J Endocrinol Metab 2019; 23(5): 545-51.
[http://dx.doi.org/10.4103/ijem.IJEM_159_19] [PMID: 31803595]

[27]   Hamid Mehmood Z-T-N, Papandreou D. An updated mini review of vitamin D and obesity: adipogenesis and inflammation state. Open Access Maced J Med Sci 2016; 4(3): 526-32.
[http://dx.doi.org/10.3889/oamjms.2016.103] [PMID: 27703587]

[28]   Wimalawansa SJ. Associations of vitamin D with insulin resistance, obesity, type 2 diabetes, and metabolic syndrome. J Steroid Biochem Mol Biol 2018; 175: 177-89.
[http://dx.doi.org/10.1016/j.jsbmb.2016.09.017] [PMID: 27662816]

[29]   Sarkar S. Molecular crosstalk between vitamin D and non-alcoholic fatty liver disease. Explor Res Hypothesis Med. 2023, 11; 000(000): 000–000.

[30]   Rafiq S, Jeppesen PB. Insulin resistance is inversely associated with the status of vitamin D in both diabetic and non-diabetic populations. Nutrients 2021; 13(6): 1742.
[http://dx.doi.org/10.3390/nu13061742] [PMID: 34063822]

[31]   Pieńkowska A, Janicka J, Duda M, *et al.* Controversial impact of Vitamin D supplementation on reducing insulin resistance and prevention of type 2 diabetes in patients with prediabetes: A systematic review. Nutrients 2023; 15(4): 983.
[http://dx.doi.org/10.3390/nu15040983] [PMID: 36839340]

[32]   Vijay GS, Ghonge S, Vajjala SM, Palal D. Prevalence of vitamin D deficiency in type 2 diabetes mellitus patients: A cross-sectional study. Cureus 2023; 15(5): e38952.
[http://dx.doi.org/10.7759/cureus.38952] [PMID: 37313077]

[33]   Mirhosseini N, Vatanparast H, Mazidi M, Kimball SM. The effect of improved serum 25-hydroxyvitamin D status on glycemic control in diabetic patients: A meta-analysis. J Clin Endocrinol Metab 2017; 102(9): 3097-110.
[http://dx.doi.org/10.1210/jc.2017-01024] [PMID: 28957454]

[34]   Mazloomzadeh S, Karami Zarandi F, Shoghli A, Dinmohammadi H. Metabolic syndrome, its components and mortality: A population-based study. Med J Islam Repub Iran 2019; 33: 11.
[http://dx.doi.org/10.47176/mjiri.33.11] [PMID: 31086790]

[35]   Krishnamoorthy Y, Rajaa S, Murali S, Sahoo J, Kar SS. Association between anthropometric risk factors and metabolic syndrome among adults in india: A systematic review and meta-analysis of observational studies. Prev Chronic Dis 2022; 19: 210231.
[http://dx.doi.org/10.5888/pcd19.210231] [PMID: 35512304]

[36]   Abboud M, Rizk R, Haidar S, Mahboub N, Papandreou D. Association between serum vitamin D and metabolic syndrome in a sample of adults in Lebanon. Nutrients 2023; 15(5): 1129.
[http://dx.doi.org/10.3390/nu15051129] [PMID: 36904128]

[37]   Theik NWY, Raji OE, Shenwai P, *et al.* Relationship and effects of vitamin D on metabolic

Syndrome: A systematic review. Cureus 2021; 13(8): e17419.
[http://dx.doi.org/10.7759/cureus.17419] [PMID: 34589329]

[38] Lee K, Kim J. Serum vitamin D status and metabolic syndrome: a systematic review and dose-response meta-analysis. Nutr Res Pract 2021; 15(3): 329-45.
[http://dx.doi.org/10.4162/nrp.2021.15.3.329] [PMID: 34093974]

[39] Ghadieh R, Mattar Bou Mosleh J, Al Hayek S, Merhi S, El Hayek Fares J. The relationship between hypovitaminosis D and metabolic syndrome: a cross sectional study among employees of a private university in Lebanon. BMC Nutr 2018; 4(1): 36.
[http://dx.doi.org/10.1186/s40795-018-0243-x] [PMID: 32153897]

[40] Al-Dabhani K, Tsilidis KK, Murphy N, *et al.* Prevalence of vitamin D deficiency and association with metabolic syndrome in a Qatari population. Nutr Diabetes 2017; 7(4): e263-3.
[http://dx.doi.org/10.1038/nutd.2017.14] [PMID: 28394362]

[41] Introduction AR. Fertil Steril 2016; 106(1): 4-5.
[http://dx.doi.org/10.1016/j.fertnstert.2016.05.009] [PMID: 27238627]

[42] Morgante G, Darino I, Spanò A, *et al.* PCOS physiopathology and vitamin D Deficiency: Biological insights and perspectives for treatment. J Clin Med 2022; 11(15): 4509.
[http://dx.doi.org/10.3390/jcm11154509] [PMID: 35956124]

[43] Sangaraju SL, Yepez D, Grandes XA, Talanki Manjunatha R, Habib S. Cardio-metabolic disease and polycystic ovarian syndrome (PCOS): A narrative review. Cureus 2022; 14(5): e25076.
[http://dx.doi.org/10.7759/cureus.25076] [PMID: 35719759]

[44] Shi XY, Huang AP, Xie DW, Yu XL. Association of vitamin D receptor gene variants with polycystic ovary syndrome: a meta-analysis. BMC Med Genet 2019; 20(1): 32.
[http://dx.doi.org/10.1186/s12881-019-0763-5] [PMID: 30764792]

[45] Armanini D, Boscaro M, Bordin L, Sabbadin C. Controversies in the pathogenesis, diagnosis and treatment of PCOS: Focus on insulin resistance, inflammation, and hyperandrogenism. Int J Mol Sci 2022; 23(8): 4110.
[http://dx.doi.org/10.3390/ijms23084110] [PMID: 35456928]

[46] Grzesiak M. Vitamin D3 action within the ovary – an updated review. Physiol Res 2020; 371-8.
[http://dx.doi.org/10.33549/physiolres.934266]

[47] Davis EM, Peck JD, Hansen KR, Neas BR, Craig LB. Associations between vitamin D levels and polycystic ovary syndrome phenotypes. Minerva Endocrinol 2019; 44(2): 176-84.
[http://dx.doi.org/10.23736/S0391-1977.18.02824-9] [PMID: 29652114]

[48] Maktabi M, Chamani M, Asemi Z. The Effects of vitamin D supplementation on metabolic status of patients with polycystic ovary syndrome: a randomized, double-blind, placebo-controlled trial. Horm Metab Res 2017; 49(7): 493-8.
[http://dx.doi.org/10.1055/s-0043-107242] [PMID: 28679140]

[49] Zhang B, Yao X, Zhong X, Hu Y, Xu J. Vitamin D supplementation in the treatment of polycystic ovary syndrome: A meta-analysis of randomized controlled trials. Heliyon 2023; 9(3): e14291.
[http://dx.doi.org/10.1016/j.heliyon.2023.e14291] [PMID: 36942243]

[50] Cochrane KM, Bone JN, Williams BA, Karakochuk CD. Optimizing vitamin D status in polycystic ovary syndrome: a systematic review and dose–response meta-analysis. Nutr Rev 2023.
[PMID: 37769789]

[51] Reda D, Elshopakey GE, Albukhari TA, *et al.* Vitamin D3 alleviates nonalcoholic fatty liver disease in rats by inhibiting hepatic oxidative stress and inflammation *via* the SREBP-1-c/ PPARα-NF-κB/IR-S2 signaling pathway. Front Pharmacol 2023; 14: 1164512.
[http://dx.doi.org/10.3389/fphar.2023.1164512] [PMID: 37261280]

[52] Kaufmann B, Reca A, Wang B, Friess H, Feldstein AE, Hartmann D. Mechanisms of nonalcoholic fatty liver disease and implications for surgery. Langenbecks Arch Surg 2021; 406(1): 1-17.

   [http://dx.doi.org/10.1007/s00423-020-01965-1] [PMID: 32833053]

[53] Jarukamjorn K, Jearapong N, Pimson C, Chatuphonprasert W. A high-fat, high-fructose diet induces antioxidant imbalance and increases the risk and progression of nonalcoholic fatty liver disease in mice. Scientifica (Cairo) 2016; 2016: 1-10.
   [http://dx.doi.org/10.1155/2016/5029414] [PMID: 27019761]

[54] Barchetta I, Cimini FA, Cavallo MG. Vitamin D and metabolic dysfunction-associated fatty liver disease (MAFLD): An update. Nutrients 2020; 12(11): 3302.
   [http://dx.doi.org/10.3390/nu12113302] [PMID: 33126575]

[55] Liu Y, Wang M, Xu W, *et al.* Active vitamin D supplementation alleviates initiation and progression of nonalcoholic fatty liver disease by repressing the p53 pathway. Life Sci 2020; 241: 117086.
   [http://dx.doi.org/10.1016/j.lfs.2019.117086] [PMID: 31756344]

[56] Sangouni AA, Ghavamzadeh S, Jamalzehi A. A narrative review on effects of vitamin D on main risk factors and severity of non-alcoholic fatty liver disease. Diabetes Metab Syndr 2019; 13(3): 2260-5.
   [http://dx.doi.org/10.1016/j.dsx.2019.05.013] [PMID: 31235166]

[57] Chen X, Zhao Y, Zhang R, Zhao Y, Dai L. The effect of vitamin D supplementation on some metabolic parameters in patients with nonalcoholic fatty liver disease: A systematic review and meta-analysis of 8 RCTs. Medicine (Baltimore) 2023; 102(42): e35717.
   [http://dx.doi.org/10.1097/MD.0000000000035717] [PMID: 37861495]

[58] Delrue C, Speeckaert R, Delanghe JR, Speeckaert MM. The role of vitamin D in diabetic nephropathy: A translational approach. Int J Mol Sci 2022; 23(2): 807.
   [http://dx.doi.org/10.3390/ijms23020807] [PMID: 35054991]

[59] Huang HY, Lin TW, Hong ZX, Lim LM. Vitamin D and diabetic kidney disease. Int J Mol Sci 2023; 24(4): 3751.
   [http://dx.doi.org/10.3390/ijms24043751] [PMID: 36835159]

[60] Krairittichai U, Mahannopkul R, Bunnag S. An open label, randomized controlled study of oral calcitriol for the treatment of proteinuria in patients with diabetic kidney disease. J Med Assoc Thai 2012; 95 (Suppl. 3): S41-7.
   [PMID: 22619886]

[61] Barzegari M, Sarbakhsh P, Mobasseri M, *et al.* The effects of vitamin D supplementation on lipid profiles and oxidative indices among diabetic nephropathy patients with marginal vitamin D status. Diabetes Metab Syndr 2019; 13(1): 542-7.
   [http://dx.doi.org/10.1016/j.dsx.2018.11.008] [PMID: 30641762]

[62] Ahmadi N, Mortazavi M, Iraj B, Askari G. Whether vitamin D3 is effective in reducing proteinuria in type 2 diabetic patients? J Res Med Sci 2013; 18(5): 374-7.
   [PMID: 24174939]

[63] Tiryaki Ö, Usalan C, Sayiner ZA. Vitamin D receptor activation with calcitriol for reducing urinary angiotensinogen in patients with type 2 diabetic chronic kidney disease. Ren Fail 2016; 38(2): 222-7.
   [http://dx.doi.org/10.3109/0886022X.2015.1128250] [PMID: 26707134]

[64] Thethi TK, Bajwa MA, Ghanim H, *et al.* Effect of paricalcitol on endothelial function and inflammation in type 2 diabetes and chronic kidney disease. J Diabetes Complications 2015; 29(3): 433-7.
   [http://dx.doi.org/10.1016/j.jdiacomp.2015.01.004] [PMID: 25633573]

[65] Munisamy S, Daud KM, Mokhtar SS, Rasool AHG. Effects of 1α-Calcidol (Alfacalcidol) on microvascular endothelial function, arterial stiffness, and blood pressure in type ii diabetic nephropathy patients. Microcirculation 2016; 23(1): 53-61.
   [http://dx.doi.org/10.1111/micc.12256] [PMID: 26749451]

[66] Liyanage G, Lekamwasam S, Weerarathna T, Liyanage C. Effect of vitamin D therapy on bone mineral density in patients with diabetic nephropathy; a randomized, double-blind placebo controlled

clinical trial. J Diabetes Metab Disord 2021; 20(1): 229-35.
[http://dx.doi.org/10.1007/s40200-021-00737-y] [PMID: 34178834]

[67] Mao L, Ji F, Liu Y, Zhang W, Ma X. Calcitriol plays a protective role in diabetic nephropathy through anti-inflammatory effects. Int J Clin Exp Med 2014; 7(12): 5437-44.
[PMID: 25664053]

[68] Kim MJ, Frankel AH, Donaldson M, *et al.* Oral cholecalciferol decreases albuminuria and urinary TGF-β1 in patients with type 2 diabetic nephropathy on established renin–angiotensin–aldosterone system inhibition. Kidney Int 2011; 80(8): 851-60.
[http://dx.doi.org/10.1038/ki.2011.224] [PMID: 21832985]

[69] Bonakdaran S, Hami M, Hatefi A. The effects of calcitriol on albuminuria in patients with type-2 diabetes mellitus. Saudi J Kidney Dis Transpl 2012; 23(6): 1215-20.
[PMID: 23168851]

[70] Huang Y, Yu H, Lu J, *et al.* Oral supplementation with cholecalciferol 800 IU ameliorates albuminuria in Chinese type 2 diabetic patients with nephropathy. PLoS One 2012; 7(11): e50510.
[http://dx.doi.org/10.1371/journal.pone.0050510] [PMID: 23209764]

[71] Sharma P, Rani N, Gangwar A, Singh R, Kaur R, Upadhyaya K. Diabetic neuropathy: A repercussion of vitamin D deficiency. Curr Diabetes Rev 2023; 19(6): e170822207592.
[http://dx.doi.org/10.2174/1573399819666220817121551] [PMID: 35980059]

[72] Kinesya E, Santoso D, Gde Arya N, *et al.* Vitamin D as adjuvant therapy for diabetic foot ulcers: Systematic review and meta-analysis approach. Clin Nutr ESPEN 2023; 54: 137-43.
[http://dx.doi.org/10.1016/j.clnesp.2023.01.011] [PMID: 36963855]

[73] Iqhrammullah M, Duta TF, Alina M, *et al.* Role of lowered level of serum vitamin D on diabetic foot ulcer and its possible pathomechanism: A systematic review, meta-analysis, and meta-regression. Diabetes Epidemiol Manage 2024; 13: 100175.
[http://dx.doi.org/10.1016/j.deman.2023.100175]

[74] Todorova AS, Jude EB, Dimova RB, *et al.* Vitamin D status in a bulgarian population with type 2 diabetes and diabetic foot ulcers. Int J Low Extrem Wounds 2022; 21(4): 506-12.
[http://dx.doi.org/10.1177/1534734620965820] [PMID: 33094656]

[75] Priyanto MH, Legiawati L, Saldi SRF, Yunir E, Miranda E. Comparison of vitamin D levels in diabetes mellitus patients with and without diabetic foot ulcers: An analytical observational study in Jakarta, Indonesia. Int Wound J 2023; 20(6): 2028-36.
[http://dx.doi.org/10.1111/iwj.14066] [PMID: 36647686]

[76] Zubair M, Malik A, Meerza D, Ahmad J. 25-Hydroxyvitamin D [25(OH)D] levels and diabetic foot ulcer: Is there any relationship? Diabetes Metab Syndr 2013; 7(3): 148-53.
[http://dx.doi.org/10.1016/j.dsx.2013.06.008] [PMID: 23953180]

[77] Tiwari S, Pratyush DD, Gupta B, *et al.* Prevalence and severity of vitamin D deficiency in patients with diabetic foot infection. Br J Nutr 2013; 109(1): 99-102.
[http://dx.doi.org/10.1017/S0007114512000578] [PMID: 22715859]

[78] Najafipour F, Aghamohammadza N, Zonouz NR, Houshyar J. Role of serum vitamin D level in progression of diabetic foot Ulcer. Journal of Clinical and Diagnostic Research 2019.
[http://dx.doi.org/10.7860/JCDR/2019/39974.12689]

[79] Afarideh M, Ghanbari P, Noshad S, Ghajar A, Nakhjavani M, Esteghamati A. Raised serum 25-hydroxyvitamin D levels in patients with active diabetic foot ulcers. Br J Nutr 2016; 115(11): 1938-46.
[http://dx.doi.org/10.1017/S0007114516001094] [PMID: 27153203]

[80] Tiwari S, Pratyush DD, Gupta SK, Singh SK. Vitamin D deficiency is associated with inflammatory cytokine concentrations in patients with diabetic foot infection. Br J Nutr 2014; 112(12): 1938-43.
[http://dx.doi.org/10.1017/S0007114514003018] [PMID: 25331710]

[81] Lin J, Mo X, Yang Y, Tang C, Chen J. Association between vitamin D deficiency and diabetic foot

ulcer wound in diabetic subjects: A meta-analysis. Int Wound J 2023; 20(1): 55-62.
[http://dx.doi.org/10.1111/iwj.13836] [PMID: 35567425]

[82]   Wang F, Zhou L, Zhu D, Yang C. A Retrospective analysis of the relationship between 25-OH-Vitamin D and diabetic foot ulcer. Diabetes Metab Syndr Obes 2022; 15: 1347-55.
[http://dx.doi.org/10.2147/DMSO.S358170] [PMID: 35535217]

[83]   Tiwari S, Pratyush DD, Gupta SK, Singh SK. Association of vitamin D with macrophage migration inhibitory factor and interleukin-8 in diabetic foot infection. Chronicle of Diabetes Research and Practice 2022; 1(1): 9-13.
[http://dx.doi.org/10.4103/cdrp.cdrp_6_21]

[84]   Dai J, Yu M, Chen H, Chai Y. Association between serum 25-OH-Vitamin D and diabetic foot ulcer in patients with type 2 diabetes. Front Nutr 2020; 7: 109.
[http://dx.doi.org/10.3389/fnut.2020.00109] [PMID: 32984392]

CHAPTER 4

Vitamin D and Cardiovascular Diseases

May Ali[1,*], **Alyaa Masaad**[1] and **Dimitrios Papandreou**[1]

[1] *Department of Clinical Nutrition and Dietetics, College of Health Sciences, University of Sharjah, Sharjah, UAE*

Abstract: Vitamin D is an essential micronutrient crucial for various physiological functions in humans, notably impacting calcium metabolism, skeletal integrity, immune response, and cellular proliferation and differentiation. While predominantly synthesized through sunlight exposure, dietary intake, and supplementation also contribute to its availability. Vitamin D deficiency has been implicated as a potential risk factor for atherosclerosis, cardiorespiratory distress, and cardiovascular diseases (CVDs), including sudden cardiac death, hypertension, and stroke. Observational studies have indicated an inverse correlation between circulating vitamin D levels and the incidence of CVDs; however, causality remains ambiguous. Some evidence suggests a potential cardioprotective effect of vitamin D supplementation, however, further investigation is warranted to elucidate its precise role in cardiovascular health. This review aims to comprehensively present existing literature on the relationship between vitamin D status and CVDs.

Keywords: Atherosclerosis, Supplement, Cardiovascular disease, Hypertension, Vitamin D.

INTRODUCTION

Cardiovascular disease (CVD) is a widespread and complex group of conditions that affect the heart and blood vessels. It encompasses a range of disorders, including coronary artery disease, heart failure, stroke, and peripheral artery disease, among others [1]. CVD is a leading cause of morbidity and mortality worldwide, posing a significant public health challenge [2]. It claims the highest number of lives annually, resulting in 17.9 million deaths each year with heart attacks and strokes accounting for 85% of the total number [1].

In recent years, researchers have been increasingly exploring the relationship between vitamin D and cardiovascular health. This relationship is multifaceted,

* **Corresponding author May Ali:** Department of Clinical Nutrition and Dietetics, College of Health Sciences, University of Sharjah, Sharjah, UAE; E-mails: U23102372@sharjah.ac.ae, mayaly.dbx@gmail.com

Dimitrios Papandreou (Ed.)
All rights reserved-© 2024 Bentham Science Publishers

involving various mechanisms that affect the risk, development, and progression of CVDs. This is because almost all cells in the body, including cardiac and smooth muscle cells, express vitamin D receptors (VDRs) and are affected by their signalling [3].

One of the proposed mechanisms of vitamin D's role in calcium regulation starts from its absorption to regulating its function in the body. Calcium is essential for proper muscle contractions among other functions. Concerning the cardiovascular system, calcitriol ensures the transport of calcium intracellularly in varying concentrations for proper and rhythmic smooth muscle contractions. Imbalances in calcium handling, due to vitamin D deficiency, may lead to cardiac arrhythmias among other cardiovascular conditions [4].

Another mechanism involves the regulation of blood pressure through the renin-angiotensin-aldosterone system (RAAS). While RAAS is crucial for blood pressure homeostasis, its overactivation is the primary mechanism for the pathogenesis of hypertension [5]. Vitamin D is needed to help tightly regulate this system and prevent the prognosis of hypertension. Therefore, vitamin D deficiency has been associated with an increased risk of hypertension among other CVD [5] as will be elucidated later in the chapter.

An additional important pathophysiological mechanism is vitamin D's role in anti-inflammation. Vitamin D has been shown to reduce inflammation by activating antithrombotic and vasodilator genes and decreasing low-density lipoprotein (LDL) oxidization increasing the risk of plaque formation or atherosclerosis [6, 7].

With the growing body of evidence supporting the intricate relationship between vitamin D and cardiovascular health, this chapter aims to explore the current state of knowledge and highlight the key findings from research in this area linking vitamin D deficiency with sudden cardiac death, strokes, and CVD comorbidities including dyslipidemia, hypertension, and atherosclerosis.

Vitamin D and Cardiorespiratory Fitness

Examining the connection between vitamin D and its effect on cardiovascular health demonstrated mixed results in the previous decades. The latest reviews of this connection note that vitamin D deficiency harms the overall fitness of the CV system. For instance, it has been shown that the prevalence of vitamin D deficiency was higher in individuals with CVD compared with those without CVD [2]. Low vitamin D levels are persistent worldwide where estimates for the prevalence indicate percentages of 24% in the United States, and 37% in Canada, while in Europe, approximately 40% of residents are deficient, with over 10%

being severely deficient [8]. Such high numbers of people experiencing a lack of this vitamin are often connected to the increasing issues in cardiorespiratory systems.

Inadequate levels of vitamin D are also negatively related to the risk of developing cardiovascular problems in the future possibly through the immune system pathway although the vitamin's specific effect is unknown. For instance, vitamin D promotes immune tolerance and improves the responses from the immune system through T cell differentiation and suppression of T helper 1 and T helper 17 cells [9]. Vitamin D's presence in vascular muscle cells and cardiomyocytes is essential for cardiorespiratory fitness. Simultaneously, trials attempting to investigate the direct effect of adding supplements of vitamin D into the diet of both healthy individuals and people with CVD or hypertension (HTN) do not yield positive results.

Vitamin D and Sudden Cardiac Death (SCD) and Cardiovascular Mortality

Sudden cardiac death (SCD) is defined as a death due to a cardiovascular cause within 1 hour of the onset of symptoms [10]. Every year, 1 out of every 7.4 people die from out-of-hospital SCD in the US [11]. Although infrequent, SCD ranks as the primary non-traumatic cause of death among young athletes. The occurrence ranges between 0.47 – 1.21 per 100,000 persons among young athletes (≤35 years) and 6.64 per 100,000 persons among older athletes (>35 years) [12].

SCDs exhibit a circadian pattern as well, with a peak between 6 am and noon, and a smaller peak occurring in the late afternoon. Moreover, the overall rate of sudden cardiac death is higher on Mondays [13].

Acknowledging the complex and the heterogenous relationship between vitamin D and cardiovascular function, research has been looking into using serum vitamin D as a potential biomarker for SCD and possibly CVD [14, 15]. A recent meta-analysis of cohort studies showed a significant relationship between low circulating vitamin D levels and the risk of SCD and cardiovascular mortality among the healthy population and population with pre-existing comorbidities including CVD and chronic kidney disease with an overall hazard ratio of 1.84, 1.58, and 1.81, respectively [14]. There was one study included in the meta-analysis that looked at the risk of SCD and cardiovascular mortality rates among diabetic patients and that showed an overall HR of 1.90 [14].

Vitamin D and Ischemic Stroke Risk and Prognosis

Strokes are the second leading cause of death worldwide and the first leading cause of disability [16]. The probability of experiencing a stroke during one's lifetime has surged by 50% in the past 17 years, and the current estimate suggests that 1 in 4 individuals will encounter a stroke at some point in their lives [17]. The most prevalent type of strokes are ischemic strokes where the main contributor is atherosclerosis. According to the American Heart Association, forecasts indicate that the occurrence rate of ischemic strokes is set to rise across all sexes, age groups, and socio-demographic categories in certain countries between 2020 and 2030 [18]. Many studies have tried to examine the relationship between vitamin D and CVD.

Observational Studies

A meta-analysis published in 2019 showcasing 9 prospective studies, with the participants mainly being American or European, concluded that vitamin D serum level and intake are inversely associated with the risk of stroke or ischemic stroke. The performed dose-response analysis reported a non-linear association between vitamin D serum level and the risk of stroke. The risk of stroke decreased to the lowest point when vitamin D serum levels were 50 ng/ml (125 nmol/L) and when vitamin D intake was 12 ug/day [19]. In another recent meta-analysis that included 20 prospective studies and 1 case study conducted on Caucasian subjects, the authors reported an increased risk of stroke or ischemic stroke in correlation with low vitamin D serum levels [20].

Vitamin D serum levels have also been studied in correlation with stroke recurrence [21, 22]. The accumulative risk for stroke survivors to develop a recurrence increases progressively at 30 days, with 3.1%, and ten years, with 39.2% [23]. A dose-response meta-analysis included 4 prospective studies that reported a progressive inverse relationship between vitamin D serum level and the risk of stroke recurrence. Furthermore, a non-linear dose-response association was reported with the highest risk associated with a vitamin D serum level of ≤ 8.5 ng/ml (21.25 nmol/L) and the lowest risk associated with a serum level of 28.1 ng/ml (70.25 nmol/L) [22]. The analysis also reported a decrease in stroke recurrence risk if the patient had a vitamin D serum level ≥ 9.3 ng/ml (23.25 nmol/L) upon their first stroke [22].

The prognosis of cases prior to a stroke incident was also studied in relation to vitamin D serum levels. A meta-analysis showcasing prospective and retrospective studies reported an inverse association between low serum levels of vitamin D and poor prognosis in stroke patients. Patients with the lowest vitamin D serum levels increased the risk of poor functional outcomes, all-cause mortality, and risk of recurrent strokes by 1.86 folds, 3.56 folds, and 5.49 folds, respectively [21]. With these conclusions, the authors have suggested that vitamin D serum levels can be used as a biomarker for the prognosis after strokes [21].

Multiple pathophysiological mechanisms have been proposed to explain this association, such are the effects of vitamin D on RAAS [19, 21], autoimmune-inflammatory responses [19, 21, 22], cell differentiation and cell growth [22], and the prevention of secondary hyperparathyroidism [19], which all contribute to overall inflammation increasing the risk of atherosclerosis and therefore the risk of ischemic strokes.

Atherosclerosis

Atherosclerosis is a chronic disease defined by inflammation and arterial plaque formation. The connection between this condition and vitamin D levels lies in the role of the steroid hormone on the fitness of the cardiovascular system and other related issues, such as hypertension, dyslipidemia, excessive weight gain, insulin resistance, and more [24]. As noted above, cell differentiation promoted by vitamin D supports vascular smooth muscle cells, which prevents the thickening of the heart muscle walls and calcification of arteries [9]. Therefore, it can be derived that the hormone indirectly affects the risks of atherosclerosis by promoting a healthy heart, although direct connections between the two concepts are still under investigation.

Low-Grade Inflammation

The anti-inflammatory effect of sufficient vitamin D levels is related to its immune system support. The physiology of vitamin D described previously demonstrates the impact of this hormone on the differentiation of T cells. In the immune system, Tregs are cells that are responsible for effective immune responses and reduced inflammation [9]. Thus, the differentiation of Treg cells induced by vitamin D leads to suppressed inflammation of the arterial walls and reduced progression or development of atherosclerosis [9]. In contrast, vitamin D has a suppressive effect on T1 and T17 helper cell differentiation. These cells are responsible for inducing inflammatory processes, resulting in the increased risk of plaque creation in the arteries [9]. By reducing their production, the vitamin also decreases inflammation and promotes cardiovascular health. As a result, vitamin D acts in two major ways: a) by promoting the proliferation of anti-inflammatory cells and b) by inhibiting the activity of pro-inflammatory cells in the system, resulting in a balanced immune system response and plaque stability.

Dyslipidemia

Another process related to cardiovascular health and vitamin D is the concentration of lipids in the body. Dyslipidemia is a significant factor contributing to atherosclerosis and other CVDs, such as increased cholesterol, LDL, and triglycerides and reduced high-density lipoproteins [25]. This condition contributes to atherosclerosis by aiding in cholesterol accumulation in white cells and the suppression of the immune system [24]. Furthermore, dyslipidemia increases the risk of atheromatous plaque formation in arterial walls due to the high concentration of LDL in the blood.

The presence of vitamin D has been found to combat the effects of dyslipidemia on the cardiovascular system. In particular, the hormone regulates the levels of LDL and reduces the process of foam cell formation from white cells and cholesterol [9]. The fat-soluble vitamin decreases the risk of dyslipidemia and is shown to be a marker of decreased LDL and increased HDL in blood [25]. By regulating serum cholesterol, vitamin D benefits the cardiovascular system. The deficiency, in turn, exposes one to the exacerbating factors that increase the risk of plaque formation.

Hypertension in Adults and Children

Another major issue that is potentially influenced by vitamin D is hypertension (HTN). Even though commonly associated with older age, hypertension in children has been an area of concern in recent years. This widespread prevalence in both groups has ignited abundant research on whether they are connected [26]. Nonetheless, similar to other cardiovascular conditions, the relation between HTN and vitamin D deficiency is inconclusive. HTN risks are affected by the state of endothelium and its activity. Narrow arterial walls that are caused by endothelial dysfunction lead to reduced blood flow [27]. As a result, systolic and diastolic pressure is increased, and HTN develops if there is consistently high pressure.

Numerous studies have established a correlation between endothelial function and vitamin D deficiency, emphasizing the role of vitamin D in regulating HTN risk. One suggested mechanism for this association is the activation of the renin-angiotensin-aldosterone system (RAAS) by vitamin D. This activation aids in maintaining a balanced electrolyte level essential for optimal endothelial performance [28]. A connection between the deficiency of vitamin D and HTN is evident in research, but the correlation between the two concepts is unclear [29]. Several research data demonstrate that polymorphism in the vitamin D receptor gene may be responsible for making people susceptible to hypertension [30, 31].

In a recent systematic review led by [32], an examination of observational studies was conducted. The results indicated that, while one prospective cohort study suggested an inverse correlation between vitamin D levels and systolic blood pressure (BP), leading to an increased likelihood of developing hypertension a decade later, the majority of the reviewed studies did not support such a connection between vitamin D and systolic BP. The review underscores the varied methodologies employed in these studies and emphasizes concerns regarding the flawed assessment of blood pressure. The authors advocate for the necessity of long-term standardized studies to gain a more comprehensive understanding of the relationship between vitamin D and hypertension.

Overall, studies considering vitamin D levels do not consistently find a significant change in blood pressure or a direct effect of deficiency on hypertension risks.

VITAMIN D SUPPLEMENTATION

Protective Doses for Healthy Individuals

The global prevalence of vitamin D deficiency raises the question of whether healthy individuals should take supplements of vitamin D to prevent the risks of CVD later on in life. Similar to other areas of investigation, the recommendations for using increased doses of vitamin D for conditions unrelated to musculoskeletal health are mixed. The presence of deficiency should be addressed – if a person's vitamin D level is below 30 nmol/l, they should take supplements and increase the presence of foods with high vitamin D in their diet [8]. Nonetheless, studies considering the impact of increased vitamin D consumption in adults without cardiovascular conditions or severe vitamin deficiency do not demonstrate any positive results in protecting them against CVD risk in the future [8, 27].

Data on Supplementation for Individuals with CVDs

The plethora of observational studies drawing an association between vitamin D deficiency and the risk of CVD prompted many clinical studies to test the validity of using vitamin D supplementation as a preventative measure or therapy against CVD, and the results were inconclusive. Supplementation of vitamin D has been found to lower blood pressure in elderly individuals with HTN and vitamin D deficiency [29]. Furthermore, people with obesity, vitamin D deficiency, and hypertension may benefit from supplements and see a reduction in both diastolic and systolic blood pressure [26]. Increased intake of vitamin D may also impact the lipid levels in the blood and aid in reducing the risks of plaque formation in people with CVD [8, 25, 33]. Some data demonstrates the effects of adequate vitamin D levels in reducing mortality risk while limiting the impact of other factors contributing to CVDs [24, 34]. Nevertheless, vitamin D supplementation cannot be recommended for preventing or mitigating the effects of cardiovascular conditions due to differing outcomes of randomized studies, however, correcting vitamin D levels, as an early intervention, with proper sunlight exposure can be an optimal strategy [35].

CONCLUSION

The role of vitamin D in health is indisputable – the steroid hormone affects many parts of the body and plays a role in the musculoskeletal, cardiovascular, and immune systems. The deficiency of this vitamin is a global problem that is present in all age groups, ethnicities, and genders. The metabolic and pathophysiological processes reveal the ubiquitous nature of vitamin D in the differentiation of cells and the regulation of immune functions. Nonetheless, the direct link between vitamin D deficiency and cardiovascular health has not been justified, although many studies demonstrate that the two conditions often are interrelated and coincide. Vitamin D deficiency is connected to heart health and can predict atherosclerosis, increased inflammation, dyslipidemia, and hypertension. Therefore, increasing vitamin D levels in individuals with such conditions can yield positive results. However, healthy individuals do not benefit from increased vitamin intake as the latter has not been found to prevent the development of CVDs.

REFERENCES

[1]   Zhu YB, Li ZQ, Ding N, Yi HL. The association between vitamin D receptor gene polymorphism and susceptibility to hypertension: a meta-analysis. Eur Rev Med Pharmacol Sci 2019; 23(20): 9066-74. [PMID: 31696497]

[2]   Zhang D, Cheng C, Wang Y, *et al.* Effect of vitamin D on blood pressure and hypertension in the general population: an update meta-analysis of cohort studies and randomized controlled trials. Prev Chronic Dis 2020; 17: 190307. [http://dx.doi.org/10.5888/pcd17.190307] [PMID: 31922371]

[3]   World Health Organization. Cardiovascular diseases (CVDs). 2021; Available at: https://www.who.int/news-room/fact-sheets/detail/cardiovascular-diseases-(cvds)

[4]   Vergatti A, Abate V, Zarrella A, *et al.* 25-Hydroxy-vitamin D and risk of recurrent stroke: A dose response meta-analysis. Nutrients 2023; 15(3): 512. [http://dx.doi.org/10.3390/nu15030512] [PMID: 36771220]

[5]   Surdu AM, Pînzariu O, Ciobanu DM, *et al.* Vitamin D and its role in the lipid metabolism and the development of atherosclerosis. Biomedicines 2021; 9(2): 172. [http://dx.doi.org/10.3390/biomedicines9020172] [PMID: 33572397]

[6]   Su C, Jin B, Xia H, Zhao K. Association between Vitamin D and Risk of Stroke: A PRISMA-Compliant Systematic Review and Meta-Analysis. Eur Neurol 2021; 84(6): 399-408. [http://dx.doi.org/10.1159/000517584] [PMID: 34325429]

[7]   Shi H, Chen H, Zhang Y, *et al.* 25-Hydroxyvitamin D level, vitamin D intake, and risk of stroke: A dose–response meta-analysis. Clin Nutr 2020; 39(7): 2025-34. [http://dx.doi.org/10.1016/j.clnu.2019.08.029] [PMID: 31530422]

[8]   Sharba ZF, Shareef RH, Abd BA, Hameed EN. Association between dyslipidemia and vitamin D deficiency: a cross-sectional study. Folia Med (Plovdiv) 2021; 63(6): 965-9. [http://dx.doi.org/10.3897/folmed.63.e62417] [PMID: 35851223]

[9]   Savolainen L, Timpmann S, Mooses M, *et al.* Vitamin D supplementation has no impact on cardiorespiratory fitness, but improves inflammatory status in vitamin D deficient young men engaged in resistance training. Nutrients 2022; 14(24): 5302. [http://dx.doi.org/10.3390/nu14245302] [PMID: 36558461]

[10] Risgaard B, Winkel BG, Jabbari R, *et al.* Sports-related sudden cardiac death in a competitive and a noncompetitive athlete population aged 12 to 49 years: Data from an unselected nationwide study in Denmark. Heart Rhythm 2014; 11(10): 1673-81.
[http://dx.doi.org/10.1016/j.hrthm.2014.05.026] [PMID: 24861446]

[11] Pu L, Wang L, Zhang R, Zhao T, Jiang Y, Han L. Projected global trends in ischemic stroke incidence, deaths and disability-adjusted life years from 2020 to 2030. Stroke 2023; 54(5): 1330-9.
[http://dx.doi.org/10.1161/STROKEAHA.122.040073] [PMID: 37094034]

[12] Papandreou D. Impact of vitamin D on cardiovascular disease - mini review. Perspect Agric Vet Sci Nutr Nat Resour 2016; 11(45): 1-2.

[13] Oberoi D, Mehrotra V, Rawat A. "Vitamin D" as a profile marker for cardiovascular diseases. Ann Card Anaesth 2019; 22(1): 47-50.
[http://dx.doi.org/10.4103/aca.ACA_66_18] [PMID: 30648679]

[14] Nunes IFOC, Cavalcante AACM, Alencar MVOB, *et al.* Meta-analysis of the association between the rs228570 vitamin D receptor gene polymorphism and arterial hypertension risk. Adv Nutr 2020; 11(5): 1211-20.
[http://dx.doi.org/10.1093/advances/nmaa076] [PMID: 32597926]

[15] Liu H, Wang J, Xu Z. Prognostic utility of serum 25-hydroxyvitamin D in patients with stroke: a meta-analysis. J Neurol 2020; 267(11): 3177-86.
[http://dx.doi.org/10.1007/s00415-019-09599-0] [PMID: 31705290]

[16] Latic N, Erben RG. Vitamin D and cardiovascular disease, with emphasis on hypertension, atherosclerosis, and heart failure. Int J Mol Sci 2020; 21(18): 6483.
[http://dx.doi.org/10.3390/ijms21186483] [PMID: 32899880]

[17] Kong SY, Jung E, Hwang S, *et al.* Circulating vitamin D level and risk of sudden cardiac death and cardiovascular mortality: A dose-response meta-analysis of prospective studies. J Korean Med Sci 2023; 38(33): e260.
[http://dx.doi.org/10.3346/jkms.2023.38.e260] [PMID: 37605499]

[18] Khanolkar S, Hirani S, Mishra A, *et al.* Exploring the role of vitamin D in atherosclerosis and its impact on cardiovascular events: a comprehensive review. Cureus 2023; 15(7): e42470.
[http://dx.doi.org/10.7759/cureus.42470] [PMID: 37637551]

[19] Kassi E, Adamopoulos C, Basdra EK, Papavassiliou AG. Role of vitamin D in atherosclerosis. Circulation 2013; 128(23): 2517-31.
[http://dx.doi.org/10.1161/CIRCULATIONAHA.113.002654] [PMID: 24297817]

[20] Janjusevic M, Gagno G, Fluca AL, *et al.* The peculiar role of vitamin D in the pathophysiology of cardiovascular and neurodegenerative diseases. Life Sci 2022; 289: 120193.
[http://dx.doi.org/10.1016/j.lfs.2021.120193] [PMID: 34864062]

[21] He S, Hao X. The effect of vitamin D3 on blood pressure in people with vitamin D deficiency. Medicine (Baltimore) 2019; 98(19): e15284.
[http://dx.doi.org/10.1097/MD.0000000000015284] [PMID: 31083159]

[22] Hayashi M, Shimizu W, Albert CM. The spectrum of epidemiology underlying sudden cardiac death. Circ Res 2015; 116(12): 1887-906.
[http://dx.doi.org/10.1161/CIRCRESAHA.116.304521] [PMID: 26044246]

[23] Flach C, Muruet W, Wolfe C, Bhalla A, Douiri A. Risk and secondary prevention of stroke recurrence: A population-base cohort study. Stroke (1970), 2020;51(8): 2435-2444.
[http://dx.doi.org/10.1161/STROKEAHA.120.028992]

[24] Feigin VL, Brainin M, Norrving B, *et al.* World stroke organization (WSO): global stroke fact sheet 2022. 2022; 17(1): 18-29.

[25] Farapti F, Fadilla C, Yogiswara N, Adriani M. Effects of vitamin D supplementation on 25(OH)D

concentrations and blood pressure in the elderly: a systematic review and meta-analysis. F1000 Res 2020; 9: 633.
[http://dx.doi.org/10.12688/f1000research.24623.3] [PMID: 32968483]

[26]   Fanari Z, Hammami S, Hammami MB, Hammami S, Abdellatif A. Vitamin D deficiency plays an important role in cardiac disease and affects patient outcome: Still a myth or a fact that needs exploration? J Saudi Heart Assoc 2015; 27(4): 264-71.
[http://dx.doi.org/10.1016/j.jsha.2015.02.003] [PMID: 26557744]

[27]   De la Guía-Galipienso F, Martínez-Ferran M, Vallecillo N, Lavie CJ, Sanchis-Gomar F, Pareja-Galeano H. Vitamin D and cardiovascular health. Clin Nutr 2021; 40(5): 2946-57.
[http://dx.doi.org/10.1016/j.clnu.2020.12.025] [PMID: 33397599]

[28]   Choudhury S, Bae S, Ke Q, *et al.* Abnormal calcium handling and exaggerated cardiac dysfunction in mice with defective vitamin d signaling. PLoS One 2014; 9(9): e108382.
[http://dx.doi.org/10.1371/journal.pone.0108382] [PMID: 25268137]

[29]   Carbone F, Mach F, Vuilleumier N, Montecucco F. Potential pathophysiological role for the vitamin D deficiency in essential hypertension. World J Cardiol 2014; 6(5): 260-76.
[http://dx.doi.org/10.4330/wjc.v6.i5.260] [PMID: 24944756]

[30]   Benjamin EJ, Virani SS, Callaway CW, *et al.* Heart disease and stroke statistics—2018 update: A report from the american heart association. Circulation 2018; 137(12): e67-e492.
[http://dx.doi.org/10.1161/CIR.0000000000000558] [PMID: 29386200]

[31]   Barbarawi M, Kheiri B, Zayed Y, *et al.* Vitamin D supplementation and cardiovascular disease risks in more than 83 000 individuals in 21 randomized clinical trials: a meta-analysis. JAMA Cardiol 2019; 4(8): 765-76.
[http://dx.doi.org/10.1001/jamacardio.2019.1870] [PMID: 31215980]

[32]   Amrein K, Scherkl M, Hoffmann M, *et al.* Vitamin D deficiency 2.0: an update on the current status worldwide. Eur J Clin Nutr 2020; 74(11): 1498-513.
[http://dx.doi.org/10.1038/s41430-020-0558-y] [PMID: 31959942]

[33]   Allison G. Yow, Venkat Rajasurya, Sandeep Sharma statpearls sudden cardiac death. StarPearls Publishing 2022.

[34]   Abboud M, Al Anouti F, Papandreou D, Rizk R, Mahboub N, Haidar S. Vitamin D status and blood pressure in children and adolescents: a systematic review of observational studies. Syst Rev 2021; 10(1): 60.
[http://dx.doi.org/10.1186/s13643-021-01584-x] [PMID: 33618764]

[35]   World Health Organisation. World Stroke Day 2022 [Internet]. www.who.int. 2022. Available from: https://www.who.int/srilanka/news/detail/29-10-2022-world-stroke-day-2022

CHAPTER 5

Vitamin D and Irritable Bowel Syndrome

Salma Abu Qiyas[1,*], **Sheima T. Saleh**[1] and **Dimitrios Papandreou**[1]

[1] Department of Clinical Nutrition and Dietetics, College of Health Sciences, University of Sharjah, Sharjah, UAE

Abstract: Irritable bowel syndrome (IBS) is a common gastrointestinal condition characterized by abnormal bowel habits (diarrhea, constipation, or both), poor mental health, and a reduced quality of life. Although commonly diagnosed through the Rome IV criteria, a universally agreed-upon diagnostic standard for IBS is yet to be established. Several therapeutic modalities are commonly employed to treat IBS, but the lack of a distinct biomarker for the condition makes it challenging for healthcare providers to evaluate the effectiveness of treatments. Elimination diets such as the low FODMAP diet may provide benefits to patients with IBS, however, the accompanying increased risk of nutritional deficiencies may worsen the condition's symptoms. Vitamin D (VD) supplementation may reduce symptom intensity and enhance the overall quality of life for individuals with IBS through several postulated mechanisms of action, including possible influence on gut microbiota and serotonin levels. This chapter reviews the current evidence from observational studies, systematic reviews, and meta-analyses of randomized controlled trials linking VD deficiency and/or supplementation with IBS. Four observational studies found a connection between diagnosed IBS and patients' vitamin D levels, along with a correlation with symptom severity, while two studies showed contradictory results. Systematic reviews and meta-analyses suggest a positive association between vitamin D supplementation and the relief of IBS symptoms as well as improvements in mental health. Despite these encouraging results, further large-scale clinical trials are needed to establish conclusive findings and enhance clinical approaches for effectively managing IBS.

Keywords: Deficiency, Irritable bowel syndrome, Supplementation, Vitamin D.

INTRODUCTION

Irritable bowel syndrome (IBS) is a common gastrointestinal disorder that impacts 4%-10% of the global population [1]. The incidence of IBS is characterized by significant variability among different populations, as the condition tends to manifest twice as many times among women and more frequently among people under 50 [2].

* **Corresponding author Salma Abu Qiyas:** Department of Clinical Nutrition and Dietetics, College of Health Sciences, University of Sharjah, Sharjah, UAE; E-mails: U23102372@sharjah.ac.ae, sabuqiyas@gmail.com

Dimitrios Papandreou (Ed.)

Typically, patients with IBS present with gastrointestinal complaints such as abdominal pain and a change in bowel habits, presenting as diarrhea or constipation, often occurring alternately. Concurring symptoms may include indigestion, bloating, an intense urge to have a bowel movement, a sense of incomplete evacuation, chronic pelvic discomfort, migraines, and fibromyalgia [3]. Symptoms can vary widely in intensity among patients and throughout the disease course, ranging from mild to debilitating [1, 4]. Patients with IBS are more susceptible to mental health challenges such as depression and anxiety and suffer from a lower quality of life [5].

Although a clear and universally accepted diagnostic criterion for IBS has not been defined, the Rome IV criteria are most commonly used [6]. According to Rome IV criteria, IBS is diagnosed based on recurring abdominal discomfort, bloating, constipation, or diarrhea in the absence of structural or chemical changes. For a diagnosis to be made, patients should have chronic symptoms that occurred at least once per week on average in the previous three months, lasting at least six months. Based on the prevalent bowel patterns during days with irregular bowel movements, IBS can appear in one of three primary subtypes: 1) constipation-predominant IBS, 2) diarrhea-predominant IBS, and 3) mixed IBS [7, 8] (Fig. **1**).

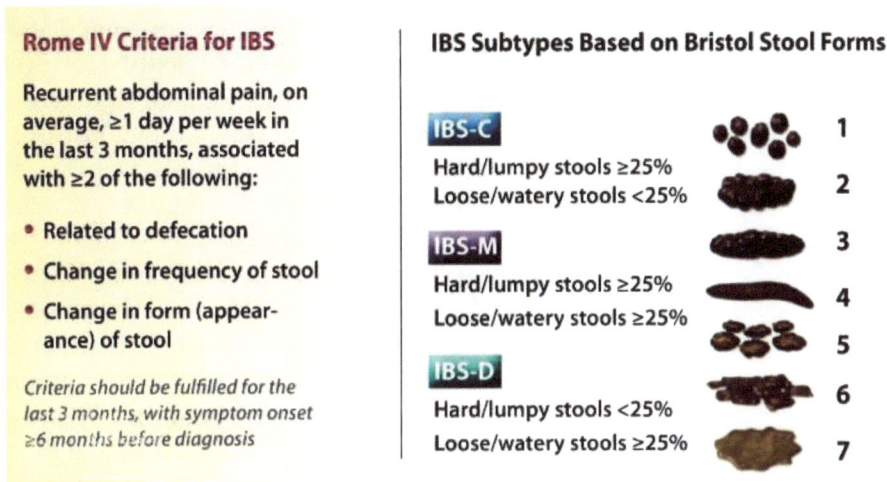

Rome IV Criteria for IBS

Recurrent abdominal pain, on average, ≥1 day per week in the last 3 months, associated with ≥2 of the following:

- Related to defecation
- Change in frequency of stool
- Change in form (appear-ance) of stool

Criteria should be fulfilled for the last 3 months, with symptom onset ≥6 months before diagnosis

IBS Subtypes Based on Bristol Stool Forms

IBS-C
Hard/lumpy stools ≥25%
Loose/watery stools <25%

IBS-M
Hard/lumpy stools ≥25%
Loose/watery stools ≥25%

IBS-D
Hard/lumpy stools <25%
Loose/watery stools ≥25%

1 2 3 4 5 6 7

Fig. (1). IBS definition and classification. (Source: Lacy *et al.* 2016).

Patients with IBS use the healthcare system more often than other gastroenterology patients. The complexity and variability of IBS presentation make treating the condition particularly challenging [9]. For instance, IBS symptoms can resemble those of other conditions like lactose or fructose intolerance, leading to a lack of response to standard treatment. Additionally, the absence of a specific biomarker for IBS complicates the assessment of treatment effectiveness for healthcare providers. Standard tests typically yield normal results, which can be frustrating for patients experiencing persistent symptoms [10].

In the initial phase and subsequent steps of the treatment plan, IBS therapy is tailored according to the most prominent symptom [11]. The first-line approach for treatment includes medications for the management of abdominal pain, cramping, constipation, and/or diarrhea. For patients suffering from significant psychological symptoms or several coinciding somatic conditions, utilizing a neuromodulator has been recommended as an initial treatment. Moreover, a diet that eliminates certain sugars linked to gastrointestinal discomfort, such as the low FODMAP diet, has been advocated as an alternative approach [12]. However, concerns over encountering symptoms after consuming particular foods may cause individuals with IBS to unnecessarily remove some foods from their diet, increasing their vulnerability to nutritional deficiencies. The culminating effects of these deficiencies may further worsen symptoms and quality of life among this group [6].

The current body of literature suggests a positive role of nutritional supplementation in the context of IBS. In particular, investigations into vitamin D supplementation have unveiled promising outcomes, notably in the reduction of symptom intensity and the enhancement of the overall quality of life for individuals affected by the condition [6]. Several mechanistic pathways have been postulated to underpin these effects. While the precise pathogenesis of IBS remains unclear, a growing body of research has suggested a link between gut dysbiosis and developing IBS, given its associations with heightened intestinal permeability, inflammatory processes, and altered neuronal activity [13]. Vitamin D supplementation appears to exert an influence on the gut microbiota, fostering an increase in beneficial bacterial strains such as Ruminococcus, Faecalibacterium, Akkermansia, Lactococcus, Coprococcus, and Bifidobacteria while concurrently reducing the prevalence of the Firmicutes microbial composition [14, 15]. These changes insinuate that vitamin D plays an immunomodulatory role by encouraging the generation of antimicrobial peptides, overseeing the maintenance of the integrity of intestinal epithelial cells, suppressing proinflammatory immune responses, and bolstering the adaptive immune system, as illustrated in Fig. (**2**) [16].

Moreover, serotonin receptors have been observed to have a pivotal role in gastrointestinal function, and their malfunction can give rise to IBS-related symptoms [17]. Vitamin D is involved in maintaining normal serotonin levels, potentially positively impacting the psychological well-being of IBS patients through its influence on brain-gut interactions. This influence may serve to mitigate symptoms of anxiety and depression [18].

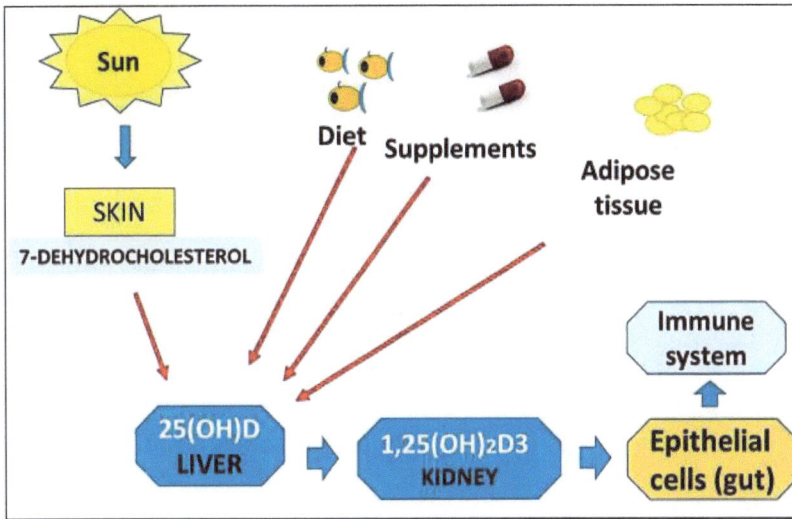

Fig. (2). Activation of 7-dehydrocholesterol in the skin occurs due to sun exposure, which undergoes further changes in the liver and kidney. Calcitriol may disrupt the integrity of epithelial cells and further the immune system. Other sources include diet and supplementation. *Adapted with permission from (Barbalho et al.,* 2019).

This chapter examines the current evidence surrounding the connection between IBS and vitamin D levels by summarizing the results of observational studies, systematic reviews, and meta-analyses of randomized controlled trials (RCTs). The discussed observational studies offer valuable information on associations between vitamin D levels and the occurrence of IBS, while the latter evaluates the impact of supplementation with vitamin D on alleviating the symptoms and enhancing the quality of life for individuals with IBS. The objective of reviewing these studies is to shed light on the potential influence of vitamin D in the treatment of IBS.

Recent Evidence of Vitamin D Supplementation in IBS

Observational Studies

Six observational studies were identified that assessed vitamin D status in patients with IBS [19 - 24].

Three retrospective case-control studies explored vitamin D levels among adults and adolescents diagnosed with IBS. The first study, conducted in Saudi Arabia, examined circulating vitamin D levels in adults with IBS as per ROME III criteria. The research comprised individuals with IBS and healthy controls, matched for age and sex (60 vs 100, respectively). Vitamin D levels were retrospectively obtained from medical records, revealing a significant difference between cases and controls. In this study, 82% of IBS cases were vitamin D deficient, as opposed to 31% in the control group (p=0.025) [19]. In the United States, another study examined the levels of vitamin D among children and adolescents diagnosed with IBS, with 55 IBS cases and 116 healthy controls. Similar results were observed, with a significantly higher percentage of vitamin D deficient subjects in cases compared to controls (50% vs. 27% respectively, p=0.001) [20].

A more recent study by Matthews *et al.* (2023) examined the levels of vitamin D and the gut microbiome makeup in adult women diagnosed with IBS and healthy controls (n=99 vs. n=62, respectively). The study found that both groups had comparable levels of vitamin D insufficiency as well as deficiency. The likelihood of having IBS was not affected by vitamin D status, and the mean levels of vitamin D were comparable between the IBS and control groups. The study revealed no correlation between plasma vitamin D levels and the diversity of the gut microbiome or the presence of specific bacteria in both the control and IBS groups [23].

A recent case report study was conducted among adults diagnosed with IBS. A total of 111 patients were provided with vitamin D supplements for 12 weeks. According to the authors, vitamin D supplementation resulted in total alleviation from IBS-related dyspepsia in 56.7% of the patients, while 36.1% reported significant improvement. The authors conclude that vitamin D supplementation could enhance dyspepsia symptoms in patients suffering from IBS [24].

Two cross-sectional studies assessed vitamin D levels and their relationship with symptom severity among adults and adolescents with IBS. The first study, conducted in South Korea, included 124 adolescents. Serum vitamin D concentration was determined by measuring 25-OHD levels using a chemiluminescent technique. Symptom severity and school absenteeism due to IBS symptoms were assessed *via* a questionnaire. Findings indicated a low mean vitamin D level among patients, with a negative relationship between vitamin D levels with symptom intensity (p = 0.022) and school absenteeism (p = 0.001). Overall, this study suggested a connection between vitamin D deficiency and symptom severity in adolescents with IBS, although limitations included a constrained study design and an unvalidated symptom severity assessment tool [21].

The second study revealed contradictory results. This study was conducted in Lebanon among adults with IBS. Vitamin D levels were measured using a chemiluminescent technique, and IBS symptoms were assessed using the Birmingham IBS scale in a sample of 230 adults. Although 67.4% of patients were deficient in vitamin D, no significant link was identified between the levels of vitamin D and the symptoms of IBS [22].

A study by Xu *et al.* used Mendelian randomization to investigate the causal association between vitamin D levels and functional gastrointestinal illnesses. The study drew on data from thousands of participants in genome-wide association studies of vitamin D and functional gastrointestinal diseases such as IBS and functional dyspepsia (n=187,028 and 194,071, respectively). The data indicated no causal relationship between vitamin D intake and functional gastrointestinal problems. However, a negative causal connection was discovered between genetically determined 25-hydroxyvitamin D levels and IBS. The incidence of IBS was reduced by approximately 16.8% for every incremental standard deviation increase in genetically determined 25-hydroxyvitamin D levels [25].

Among the reviewed observational studies, four provided evidence of an association between being diagnosed with IBS and patients' vitamin D levels, in addition to an association with symptom severity, while two presented contrasting findings. However, the findings of these studies are subject to some limitations due to their observational nature, which confines the ability to establish causality, and the relatively small sample sizes, hindering the generalizability of findings to a broader population. Moreover, while the Mendelian randomization study indicates a protective effect of serum vitamin D against IBS rather than functional dyspepsia, large-sample RCTs to comprehensively clarify the association between serum vitamin D levels and IBS are needed, given that genetic variants only explain a portion of the IBS risk variation. A summary of the discussed observational studies is provided in Table **1**.

Systematic Reviews and Meta-Analysis

Several systematic reviews published in recent years investigated the impact of regular and exclusion diets on nutritional intake in adults with IBS, as well as the potential significance of vitamin D supplementation in reducing IBS symptom severity and improving the quality of life in people with IBS. Table **2** summarizes the findings of the studies.

Table 1. A summary of observational studies on the relationship between Vitamin D and IBS.

Refs.	Study Design	Study Population	n	Relationship Between IBS and Vitamin D	Outcomes
[19]	Case-Control Study	Adults	Cases: 60 Controls: 100	Deficiency and IBS diagnosis	In contrast to 31% in the control group, 82% of cases were vitamin D deficient
[20]	Case-Control Study	Children and Adolescents	Cases: 55 Controls: 116	Deficiency and IBS diagnosis	Vitamin D levels are significantly lower in cases (50% deficient) vs. controls (27% deficient)
[21]	Cross-sectional Study	Adolescents	124	Deficiency and IBS symptoms and school absence	Low mean vitamin D (16.25 ng/mL); levels negatively associated with symptom intensity ($p=0.022$) and school absenteeism ($p=0.001$)
[24]	Case report	Adults	111	IBS-related dyspepsia and vitamin D supplementation	Total alleviation from IBS-related dyspepsia in 56.7% of the patients, while 36.1% reported significant improvement
[22]	Cross-Sectional Study	Adults	230	Deficiency and IBS symptoms	67.4% prevalence of vitamin D deficiency, no association with IBS symptoms
[23]	Case-control study	Adults (Females)	Cases: 99 Controls: 62	Deficiency and IBS symptoms	No significant difference in vitamin D deficiency (40.3% in controls and 41.4% in cases) and insufficiency (33.9% in controls and 34.3% in cases). Odds of having IBS were not significantly influenced by vitamin D status
[25]	Mendelian randomization of genome-wide associated studies from UK biobank	Adults	IBS: 187,028 Functional dyspepsia 194,071	Vitamin D level and functional gastrointestinal disorders	Genetically higher 25-hydroxyvitamin D levels were linked to a decreased risk of IBS, 16.8% reduction in incidence observed for each additional standard deviation increase in these levels

Table 2. A summary of systematic reviews and meta-analyses on vitamin D status and supplementation in IBS.

Refs.	Study Design	Studies Included	Outcomes Measured	Main Findings
[26]	Systematic Review	26 studies 12 intervention and 14 observational	Micronutrient status, dietary impact	People with IBS exhibit lower baseline vitamin B2, calcium, vitamin D, and iron levels.
[27]	Systematic Review and Meta-analysis	63 studies (intervention and observational)	Dietary intake in adults with IBS	Inadequate fiber and vitamin D intake Other macro- and micronutrient intake is unaffected Calcium is lower in adults with IBS.
[28]	Systematic Review	10 RCTs (4 IBD, 6 IBS)	Mental health outcomes (QoL, anxiety, depression)	Supplementing with vitamin D improves mental health outcomes.
[31]	Systematic Review and Meta-analysis	8 RCTs	IBS-SSS IBS-QoL	Significant improvement in IBS-SSS scores. Limited significance in IBS-QoL scores.
[32]	Systematic Review and Meta-analysis	4 RCTs	IBS-SSS IBS-QoL	Significant improvements in IBS-SSS and IBS-QoL.
[33]	Systematic Review and Meta-analysis	6 RCTs	IBS-SSS IBS-QoL Serum calcifediol	No significant difference in IBS-SSS. Favorable improvement for IBS-QoL, serum calcifediol
[34]	Systematic Review and Meta-analysis	12 RCTs	Serum vitamin D, vitamin D deficiency, IBS-SSS IBS-QoL	Low levels of vitamin D Improved IBS-QoL Effect on IBS-SSS non-significant

Two systematic reviews compared the nutrient status of IBS and non-IBS subjects. Bek *et al.* systematically analyzed data from 26 articles, consisting of 14 observational and 12 interventional studies, to investigate how micronutrient status is impacted by regular and exclusion diets in adults with IBS. Overall, their findings revealed that people with IBS exhibited lower baseline levels of a number of nutrients, including vitamin B2, D, iron, and calcium, than non-IBS subjects. Notably, exclusion diets were linked to reduced micronutrient intake, including vitamin B1, B2, iron, calcium, and zinc. These findings emphasize the importance of proper dietary management for IBS patients, potentially involving dietitian oversight to ensure nutritional adequacy [26].

In a systematic review and meta-analysis by Veraza *et al.*, nutrient intake was compared among adults with IBS vs. healthy controls. The findings revealed that individuals with IBS often fell short of recommended dietary fiber and vitamin D intake levels and had significantly lower fiber intake than controls. However, analysis revealed that IBS does not appear to have an impact on the consumption of other macro and micronutrients except for calcium, which is lower in adults with IBS than controls [27].

One systematic review by Głąbska *et al.* (2021) investigated vitamin D supplementation's impact on the mental health of people suffering from inflammatory bowel diseases (IBD) and IBS. A total of 10 RCTs were included, of which six were IBS-related. These studies evaluated diverse doses of vitamin D supplementation, comparing outcomes against placebos, with supplementation regimes extending for at least six weeks. Disease-specific quality of life, anxiety, and depression were among the mental health outcomes studied. Most studies found that vitamin D administration improved the mental health outcome measures of IBD and IBS patients, which was consistently observed despite variations in dosages and supplementation techniques [28].

The following four systematic reviews and meta-analyses were conducted to investigate the impact of supplementation on reducing symptom severity (IBS-SSS) and enhancing the quality of life scores (IBS-QoL) among individuals with IBS [29, 30].

Chong *et al.* (2022) conducted a systematic review and meta-analysis that incorporated data from eight RCTs encompassing 685 patients. The results showed IBS symptom severity scores were significantly improved post vitamin D supplementation. On the other hand, no statistical significance in IBS-QoL scores was recorded, although improvements in the scores were observed. The study highlighted certain limitations, including small sample sizes, youthful study populations, inadequate representation of ethnicities, and diverse vitamin D administration protocols. Despite these limitations, the findings suggest that vitamin D administration may be a valuable addition to the clinical management of IBS patients, given its potential efficacy and favorable safety profile [31].

Another systematic review and meta-analysis included four RCTs, including 335 participants. When compared to the placebo groups, participants receiving vitamin D supplementation showed significant improvements in IBS symptom severity scores and IBS quality of life. Specifically, the difference in scores of IBS symptom severity between the intervention and placebo groups increased significantly after the intervention. Participants who received vitamin D supplementation exhibited a more significant enhancement in both scores after intervention than those who received a placebo. The authors concluded that vitamin D supplementation may benefit people suffering from IBS [32].

Abuelazm *et al.* (2022) conducted a more recent systematic review and meta-analysis that included six RCTs totaling 616 IBS patients. According to the pooled analysis, there was no significant improvement in the primary outcome—the IBS symptom severity score—observed with either vitamin D or placebo. But when it came to enhancing secondary outcomes—namely, the quality of life for those with IBS and serum levels of calcifediol (25(OH)D)—vitamin D outperformed a placebo. The findings imply that although vitamin D may benefit secondary IBS outcomes, more clinical research is required to establish more conclusive and broadly applicable conclusions [33].

Finally, a comprehensive meta-analysis of 12 clinical trials involving 1331 IBS patients was conducted to assess the relationship between vitamin D and IBS. The primary endpoints in this study encompassed serum vitamin D levels, the risk of deficiency in IBS patients, and the IBS-SSS and QoL scores. The analysis revealed that IBS patients generally exhibit lower serum vitamin D levels. Notably, vitamin D supplementation resulted in improved IBS-QoL scores, although it did not significantly impact IBS-SSS scores [34].

In summary, the systematic reviews and meta-analyses highlight the substantial impact of dietary factors, particularly vitamin D, on individuals with IBS. Lower baseline levels of essential nutrients, especially in those following exclusion diets, underscore the importance of meticulous dietary management overseen by dietitians. Available evidence indicates a favorable association between vitamin D supplementation and the alleviation of IBS symptoms and the improvement of mental health. The evidence also suggests a positive role for vitamin D supplementation in alleviating IBS symptoms and improving mental health. Despite these promising findings, further large-scale clinical trials are emphasized to establish definitive conclusions and optimize clinical strategies for managing IBS effectively.

CONCLUSION

The comprehensive overview of IBS presented in this chapter underscores the multifaceted nature of the condition, characterized by varied symptoms, a lack of universally accepted diagnostic criteria, and the challenge of differentiating it from other gastrointestinal disorders. The therapy for IBS is diverse, ranging from medications to dietary modifications, reflecting the complex and individualized nature of its management. The focus on vitamin D supplementation emerges as a promising avenue in addressing IBS, supported by observational studies demonstrating associations between deficiency in vitamin D and IBS prevalence and severity. The systematic reviews and meta-analyses provide further insights, indicating a potential positive impact of supplementing with vitamin D on the severity of IBS symptoms and the quality of life associated with the condition. Mechanistically, the influence of vitamin D on gut microbiota and serotonin levels suggests a role in addressing the underlying factors contributing to IBS. However, the need for more extensive clinical trials is highlighted, emphasizing the importance of refining treatment strategies to enhance the overall well-being of individuals affected by IBS.

REFERENCES

[1]   Jayasinghe M, Damianos JA, Prathiraja O, *et al.* Irritable bowel syndrome: Treating the gut and brain/mind at the same time. Cureus 2023; 15(8): e43404.
        [http://dx.doi.org/10.7759/cureus.43404] [PMID: 37706135]

[2]   Algera J, Lövdahl J, Sjölund J, Tornkvist NT, Törnblom H. Managing pain in irritable bowel syndrome: current perspectives and best practice. Expert Rev Gastroenterol Hepatol 2023; 17(9): 871-81.
        [http://dx.doi.org/10.1080/17474124.2023.2242775] [PMID: 37552616]

[3]   Wilkinson JM, Gill MC. Irritable bowel syndrome: questions and answers for effective care. Am Fam Physician 2021; 103(12): 727-36.
        [PMID: 34128613]

[4]   Mayer EA, Ryu HJ, Bhatt RR. The neurobiology of irritable bowel syndrome. Mol Psychiatry 2023; 28(4): 1451-65.
        [http://dx.doi.org/10.1038/s41380-023-01972-w] [PMID: 36732586]

[5]   Zamani M, Alizadeh-Tabari S, Zamani V. Systematic review with meta-analysis: the prevalence of anxiety and depression in patients with irritable bowel syndrome. Aliment Pharmacol Ther 2019; 50(2): 132-43.
        [http://dx.doi.org/10.1111/apt.15325] [PMID: 31157418]

[6]   Radziszewska M, Smarkusz-Zarzecka J, Ostrowska L. Nutrition, physical activity and supplementation in irritable bowel syndrome. Nutrients 2023; 15(16): 3662.
        [http://dx.doi.org/10.3390/nu15163662] [PMID: 37630852]

[7]   Schmulson MJ, Drossman DA. What is new in Rome IV. J Neurogastroenterol Motil 2017; 23(2): 151-63.
        [http://dx.doi.org/10.5056/jnm16214] [PMID: 28274109]

[8]   Lacy BE, Mearin F, Chang L, *et al.* Bowel disorders. Gastroenterology. 2016; 150(6): 1393-407.
        [http://dx.doi.org/10.1053/j.gastro.2016.02.031]

[9]   Goodoory VC, Guthrie EA, Ng CE, Black CJ, Ford AC. Factors associated with lower disease-specific and generic health-related quality of life in Rome IV irritable bowel syndrome. Aliment Pharmacol Ther 2023; 57(3): 323-34.
        [http://dx.doi.org/10.1111/apt.17356] [PMID: 36544055]

[10]   Saha L. Irritable bowel syndrome: Pathogenesis, diagnosis, treatment, and evidence-based medicine. World J Gastroenterol 2014; 20(22): 6759-73.
        [http://dx.doi.org/10.3748/wjg.v20.i22.6759] [PMID: 24944467]

[11]   Aziz I, Whitehead WE, Palsson OS, Törnblom H, Simrén M. An approach to the diagnosis and management of Rome IV functional disorders of chronic constipation. Expert Rev Gastroenterol Hepatol 2020; 14(1): 39-46.
        [http://dx.doi.org/10.1080/17474124.2020.1708718] [PMID: 31893959]

[12]   Camilleri M. Diagnosis and treatment of irritable bowel syndrome: a review. JAMA 2021; 325(9): 865-77.
        [http://dx.doi.org/10.1001/jama.2020.22532] [PMID: 33651094]

[13]   Tang HY, Jiang AJ, Wang XY, *et al.* Uncovering the pathophysiology of irritable bowel syndrome by exploring the gut-brain axis: a narrative review. Ann Transl Med 2021; 9(14): 1187.
[http://dx.doi.org/10.21037/atm-21-2779] [PMID: 34430628]

[14]   Tangestani H, Boroujeni HK, Djafarian K, Emamat H, Shab-Bidar S. Vitamin D and the gut microbiota: a narrative literature review. Clin Nutr Res 2021; 10(3): 181-91.
[http://dx.doi.org/10.7762/cnr.2021.10.3.181] [PMID: 34386438]

[15]   Yu XL, Wu QQ, He LP, Zheng YF. Role of in vitamin D in irritable bowel syndrome. World J Clin Cases 2023; 11(12): 2677-83.
[http://dx.doi.org/10.12998/wjcc.v11.i12.2677] [PMID: 37214583]

[16]   Barbalho SM, Goulart RA, Araújo AC, Guiguer ÉL, Bechara MD. Irritable bowel syndrome: a review of the general aspects and the potential role of vitamin D. Expert Rev Gastroenterol Hepatol 2019; 13(4): 345-59.
[http://dx.doi.org/10.1080/17474124.2019.1570137] [PMID: 30791775]

[17]   Osman U, Latha Kumar A, Sadagopan A, *et al.* The effects of serotonin receptor type 7 modulation on bowel sensitivity and smooth muscle tone in patients with irritable bowel syndrome. Cureus 2023; 15(7): e42532.
[http://dx.doi.org/10.7759/cureus.42532] [PMID: 37637561]

[18]   Berridge MJ. Vitamin D and depression: cellular and regulatory mechanisms. Pharmacol Rev 2017; 69(2): 80-92.
[http://dx.doi.org/10.1124/pr.116.013227] [PMID: 28202503]

[19]   Khayyat Y, Attar S, Vitamin D. Vitamin D deficiency in patients with irritable bowel syndrome: does it exist? Oman Med J 2015; 30(2): 115-8.
[http://dx.doi.org/10.5001/omj.2015.25] [PMID: 25960837]

[20]   Nwosu BU, Maranda L, Candela N. Vitamin D status in pediatric irritable bowel syndrome. PLoS One 2017; 12(2): e0172183.
[http://dx.doi.org/10.1371/journal.pone.0172183] [PMID: 28192499]

[21]   Cho Y, Lee Y, Choi Y, Jeong S. Association of the vitamin D level and quality of school life in adolescents with irritable bowel syndrome. J Clin Med 2018; 7(12): 500.
[http://dx.doi.org/10.3390/jcm7120500] [PMID: 30513760]

[22]   Abboud M, Haidar S, Mahboub N, Papandreou D, Al Anouti F, Rizk R. Association between Serum Vitamin D and Irritable Bowel Syndrome Symptoms in a Sample of Adults. Nutrients 2022; 14(19): 4157.
[http://dx.doi.org/10.3390/nu14194157] [PMID: 36235809]

[23]   Matthews SW, Plantinga A, Burr R, *et al.* Exploring the role of vitamin D and the gut microbiome: A cross-sectional study of individuals with irritable bowel syndrome and healthy controls. Biol Res Nurs 2023; 25(3): 436-43.
[http://dx.doi.org/10.1177/10998004221150395] [PMID: 36624571]

[24]   Alvi H, Ali G, Iqbal S, *et al.* Role of 25-hydroxyvitamin D in irritable bowel syndrome patients. J Family Med Prim Care 2022; 11(12): 7975-8.
[http://dx.doi.org/10.4103/jfmpc.jfmpc_1336_22] [PMID: 36994062]

[25]   Xu S, Luo Q, He J, Chen X, Li S, Bai Y. Causal associations of 25-hydroxyvitamin D with functional gastrointestinal disorders: a two-sample Mendelian randomization study. Genes Nutr 2023; 18(1): 14.
[http://dx.doi.org/10.1186/s12263-023-00734-1] [PMID: 37691106]

[26]   Bek S, Teo YN, Tan XH, Fan KHR, Siah KTH. Association between irritable bowel syndrome and micronutrients: A systematic review. J Gastroenterol Hepatol 2022; 37(8): 1485-97.
[http://dx.doi.org/10.1111/jgh.15891] [PMID: 35581170]

[27]   Veraza DI, Calderon G, Jansson-Knodell C, *et al.* A systematic review and meta-analysis of diet and nutrient intake in adults with irritable bowel syndrome. Neurogastroenterol Motil 2024; 36(1): e14698.

[http://dx.doi.org/10.1111/nmo.14698] [PMID: 37897138]

[28] Głąbska D, Kołota A, Lachowicz K, *et al.* Vitamin D supplementation and mental health in inflammatory bowel diseases and irritable bowel syndrome patients: a systematic review. Nutrients 2021; 13(10): 3662.
[http://dx.doi.org/10.3390/nu13103662] [PMID: 34684663]

[29] Francis CY, Morris J, Whorwell PJ. The irritable bowel severity scoring system: a simple method of monitoring irritable bowel syndrome and its progress. Aliment Pharmacol Ther 1997; 11(2): 395-402.
[http://dx.doi.org/10.1046/j.1365-2036.1997.142318000.x] [PMID: 9146781]

[30] Drossman DA, Patrick DL, Whitehead WE, *et al.* Further validation of the IBS-QOL: a disease-specific quality-of-life questionnaire. Am J Gastroenterol 2000; 95(4): 999-1007.
[http://dx.doi.org/10.1111/j.1572-0241.2000.01941.x] [PMID: 10763950]

[31] Chong RIH, Yaow CYL, Loh CYL, *et al.* Vitamin D supplementation for irritable bowel syndrome: A systematic review and meta-analysis. J Gastroenterol Hepatol 2022; 37(6): 993-1003.
[http://dx.doi.org/10.1111/jgh.15852] [PMID: 35396764]

[32] Huang H, Lu L, Chen Y, Zeng Y, Xu C. The efficacy of vitamin D supplementation for irritable bowel syndrome: a systematic review with meta-analysis. Nutr J 2022; 21(1): 24.
[http://dx.doi.org/10.1186/s12937-022-00777-x] [PMID: 35509010]

[33] Abuelazm M, Muhammad S, Gamal M, *et al.* The effect of vitamin D supplementation on the severity of symptoms and the quality of life in irritable bowel syndrome patients: A systematic review and meta-analysis of randomized controlled trials. Nutrients 2022; 14(13): 2618.
[http://dx.doi.org/10.3390/nu14132618] [PMID: 35807798]

[34] Bin Y, Kang L, Lili Y. Vitamin D status in irritable bowel syndrome and the impact of supplementation on symptoms: a systematic review and meta-analysis. Nutrición hospitalaria: Organo oficial de la Sociedad española de nutrición parenteral y enteral. 2022; 39(5): 1144-52.

CHAPTER 6

Vitamin D and Depression

Sharfa Khaleel[1,*], Rahab Sohail[1] and **Dimitrios Papandreou[1]**

[1] Department of Clinical Nutrition and Dietetics, College of Health Sciences, University of Sharjah, Sharjah, UAE

Abstract: This chapter discusses the relationship between vitamin D and depression, shedding light on the physiological functions of the unique characteristics of vitamin D, its synthesis, and its role in extraskeletal activities apart from its established function in bone metabolism. It further delves into the global prevalence of vitamin D deficiency and the rising incidence of depression worldwide. The link between vitamin D and depression is presented emphasizing the potential roles of vitamin D in neuromuscular and immune function. The document also discusses the purported mechanisms underlying the relationship between vitamin D and depression, including neuroinflammation, imbalance in calcium homeostasis, and deficiency in neurotransmitters. Furthermore, the document presents a comprehensive review of the existing literature on the topic, citing multiple studies and reviews to support the discussed findings. It covers various aspects, including the molecular basis of vitamin D, its impact on neurobehavioral health, and its association with depressive symptoms across different age groups primarily fetal origins, children, adolescents, adults, and older adults. Many studies suggest a possible connection between depression and vitamin D insufficiency, but the exact nature of this relationship and whether the supplementation of vitamin D could effectively treat depression remains ambiguous. Given that the link between vitamin D and depression has attracted attention, further well-designed trials are needed to establish causality, elucidate the practical consequences, and address the existing discrepancies and limitations in the evidence.

Keywords: Depression, Neuroinflammation, Neurotransmitters, Supplementation, Vitamin D insufficiency.

INTRODUCTION

Vitamin D is a lipophilic vitamin playing myriad roles in human health. It shows unique characteristics that differentiate it from other vitamins; its active form functions as a steroid hormone [1]. Vitamin D displays dual functionality as it can be ingested as Vitamin D_2 as part of dietary plant origins and Vitamin D_3 as part

---

[*] **Corresponding author Sharfa Khaleel:** Department of Clinical Nutrition and Dietetics, College of Health Sciences, University of Sharjah, Sharjah, UAE; E-mails: U23102372@sharjah.ac.ae, skhaleel@sharjah.ac.ae

Dimitrios Papandreou (Ed.)
All rights reserved-© 2024 Bentham Science Publishers

of animal origin like cod liver oil, liver eggs, external supplementation, and lastly endogenous production. Synthesizing vitamin D endogenously requires contact of the skin with the sun's ultraviolet B radiation to transform 7-dehydrocholesterol into bio-active vitamin D. Progressive hydroxylation in the liver and kidneys activates vitamin D to its bio-active form - calcitriol, chemically known as 1,25-dihydroxyvitamin D_3 (1,25-$(OH)_2D_3$) [2]. In the nucleus of cells, calcitriol behaves similarly to a steroid hormone by interlinking with a vitamin D receptor (VDR) that allows it to harness its biological functions [3]. In the musculoskeletal system, vitamin D, as part of bone metabolism, governs the absorption of phosphate, magnesium, and calcium in the intestine [4]. Vitamin D deficiency comprising low serum concentrations of 25-hydroxy vitamin D (25-OHD) remains a global epidemic. A recent comprehensive analysis was conducted worldwide amongst 7.9 million subjects to assess the prevalence of the deficiency of Vitamin D, globally. Results revealed that 15.7% of the population had serum 25-OHD levels less than 30 nmol/L while 47.9% of the population had serum 25-OHD less than 50 nmol/L [5]. Apart from Vitamin D's physiological functions, numerous investigations have indicated that it could play roles in neuropsychology—such that its deficiency may be associated with various adverse mental health outcomes [6]. According to WHO, "depressive disorder (depression) is a common mental disorder that includes a depressed mood or loss of pleasure/interest in activities for a prolonged time period" [7]. Amongst mental health illnesses, depression is the most common illness worldwide [8]. The world is witnessing a steep increase in depression with incident cases having risen exponentially by almost 50% since 1990 to 2017 [9]. Nutrition and its various facets have been linked to changes in mood, behaviour, development, and treatment of mental illness. Research on the relationship between nutrition and mental health has increased over the past decade, with some findings indicating that eating a balanced diet may help prevent the development of mental disorders [10].

Mounting data implicates Vitamin D's role in numerous extra skeletal activities such as neuromuscular and immune function [6]. Furthermore, recent findings that show depressed individuals with diminished serum concentrations of vitamin D, point to a possible link between low levels of Vitamin D in the body with an elevated risk of developing depression [11].

Vitamin D and Depression Purported Mechanisms

Evidence shows that among multiple molecular mechanisms believed to be of significance in the pathology of depression, inflammation takes precedence as a critical factor [12]. Vitamin D exhibits certain pro-neurogenic, antioxidant, neuromodulatory, and anti-inflammatory characteristics that form the basis for its antidepressant and anxiolytic effects [11]. As outlined below in Fig. (**1**), certain mechanisms have been purported to modulate the link between vitamin D and depression.

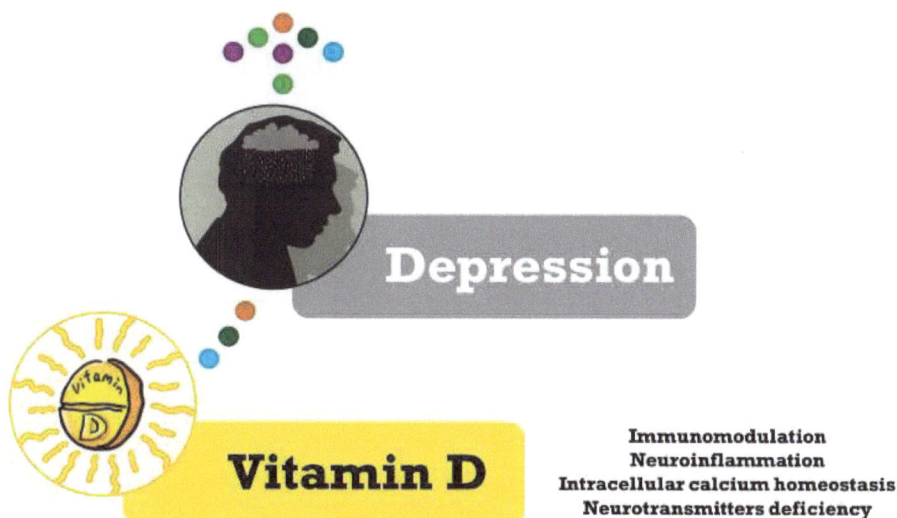

Fig. (1). Various purported mechanisms underlying Vitamin D-depression relationship.

Neuroinflammation: A Possible Mediator between Vitamin D and Depression

Neuroinflammation functions as a protective mechanism to restore the brain structure and function against physiological and infectious insults [13]. However, this protective mechanism can be detrimental and produce adverse effects in the brain when the same inflammatory process continues to be prolonged and exacerbated. Studies increasingly observe that patients with depression show elevated levels of neuroinflammatory-process-derived cytokines: IL-6, interferon-gamma (IFN-γ), tumor necrosis factor-alpha (TNF-α), which are pro-inflammatory in nature [11]. Preclinical studies on depressive rats reveal that vitamin D insufficiency could elevate inflammatory status through the production of aberrant cytokine biomarkers [14]. Thus, low serum concentrations of vitamin D could trigger inflammation. Ongoing investigations are underway to uncover the underlying mechanisms considering it still remains incompletely understood. Lowering inflammation might prove to be beneficial for patients with depression.

Imbalance in Calcium Homeostasis: A Byproduct of Vitamin D Inadequacy

There is a speculation that an inadequacy of vitamin D levels in the body could lead to a sustained elevation in Ca^{2+} levels triggering an onset of depression [15]. Calcium is required for cell signalling in the neurons, which is done by activating their inhibitory and excitatory functionalities. Excitatory neurons secrete a neurotransmitter, glutamate that triggers its targeted neuron. The neurons' collateral endings stimulate inhibitory neurons to secrete g-aminobutyric acid (GABA). Tightly regulated feedback connections between inhibitory and excitatory neurons work to ensure neuronal communication in the brain. Thus, an imbalance in calcium homeostasis could lead to disequilibrium between the two neurotransmitters namely, glutamate and GABA altering this communication, a common feature noted in depression [16]. Since Vitamin D governs intracellular calcium stores, a sufficient vitamin D level may restore calcium and neurotransmitter balance and thus positively influence depression onset.

Vitamin D, Depression, and Neurotransmitter Deficiency

It is widely acknowledged that the pathophysiology of depression can be partially attributed to deficiencies in neurotransmitters - serotonin (5-HT), dopamine (DA) and norepinephrine (NE) [17]. This is clear from the fact that antidepressant drugs, for example, tricyclic drugs, work by impeding the 5-HT and NE transporters. A deficiency in Vitamin D could impair 5-HT synthesis progressing to abnormal brain development and serotonergic neurons [18, 19]. Interestingly, multiple brain regions, particularly glial cells in the hypothalamus and neurons in the amygdala, harbor Vitamin D receptors (VDRs) [20]. Calcitriol ($1,25-(OH)_2D_3$) tethers itself to VDR in the hippocampus *via* the brain-blood barrier. These results point to the importance of vitamin D for cognitive performance, either directly or indirectly [21]. A recent study investigating the brain tissue for vitamin D-binding protein (VDBP) found that depressive patients had higher serum levels of VDBP in comparison to matched controls. Moreover, it was found that VDBP serum levels and severity of depressive symptoms were significantly correlated with each other [22]. Thus, there is compelling evidence in human and animal studies, that VDR expresses itself in the prefrontal cortex, hippocampus, and substantia nigra; these specific brain regions are known to be involved in depression. Consequently, it is speculated that lower serum concentrations of vitamin D in the substantia nigra may inhibit DA cell differentiation resulting in DA-mediated behavioural deficits. This emphasizes that low serum concentrations of vitamin D may trigger the development of depression by directly or indirectly influencing the levels of 5-HT, DA, and NE [19, 23]. Fig. (**2**) summarizes the various roles Vitamin D plays in triggering specific neuronal processes of different brain regions.

Worldwide, recent studies show that humans across all age groups: children, adolescents, adults, and the elderly, run the risk of being deficient in Vitamin D [24, 25]. Taking into account the large body of data that indicates the role of vitamin D deficiency in depression with varied functionalities, a study of Vitamin D across life span merits further study.

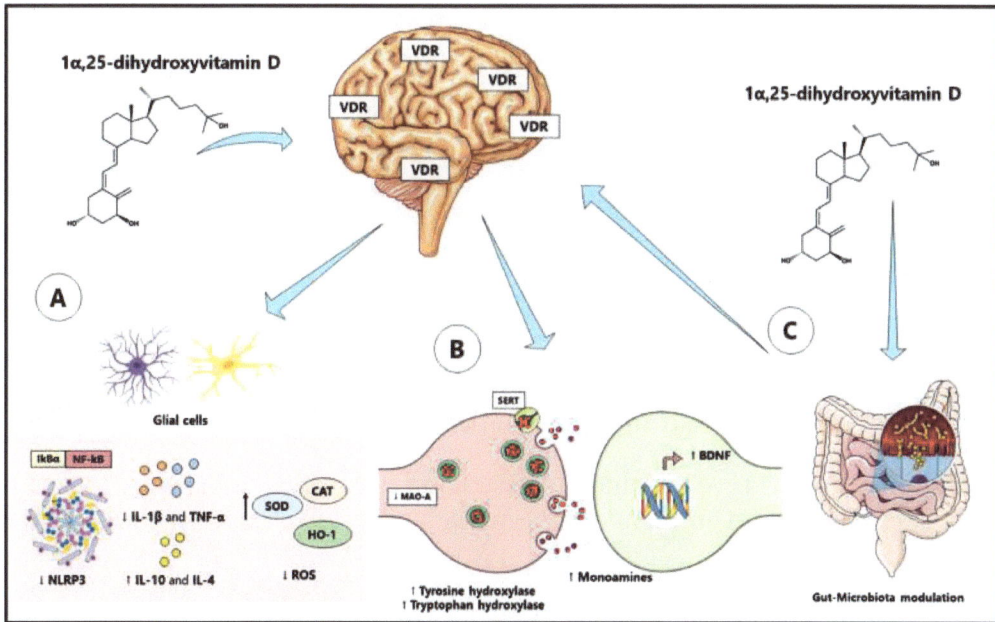

Fig. (2). Antioxidant, anti-inflammatory, and neuromodulatory properties of vitamin D. Neurons and glial cells are able to express VDR in regions such as the prefrontal cortex and hippocampus. (**A**). Modulation of Vitamin D in Gut., (**B**). Abbreviations: Abbreviations: ↓: decreased; ↑: increased; BDNF: brain-derived neurotrophic factor; CAT: catalase; HO-1: heme oxygenase-1; IL-1β: interleukin-1β; IL-4: interleukin-4; IL-10: interleukin-10; IkBα: nuclear factor of kappa light polypeptide gene enhancer in B-cells inhibitor, alpha; MAO: monoamine oxidase; NF-kB: nuclear factor kappa B; NLRP3: NOD-like receptor family pyrin domain-containing 3; ROS: reactive oxygen species; SERT: serotonin transporters; SOD: superoxide dismutase; TNF-α: tumor necrosis factor-alpha; VDR: vitamin D receptor. (**C**). Regulation of monoamines from Vitamin D. **Adapted with permission from [11, 15].**

IMPACT OF VITAMIN D ON DEPRESSION IN DIFFERENT POPULATIONS

Fetal Origins

Research suggests that deficiency in a number of micronutrients, including vitamin D, may have a role in the development of mental health issues. During gestation, deficiency of vitamin D has been extensively correlated to a reduction in the development of the fetal brain. It has also been linked to disturbances in the synthesis of brain-derived neurotrophic factors [26].

Research on both humans and animals showed that the deficiency of vitamin D during development has a significant impact on the neurobehavioral health of later offspring [27]. Moreover, according to a recent review, mother's vitamin D concentrations throughout fertilization, pregnancy, along with the period immediately before and after birth contributes to the regulation of the development of an embryo, formation of the skeletal system, as well as levels of calcium in the developing fetus. The level of vitamin D in maternal blood has an impact on the development of the nervous system, and the deficiency could increase the risk of neurological disorders [28]. A prospective study's findings demonstrated a direct relationship between a mother's vitamin D level and depression in offspring [29]. Another large prospective study found scant proof for an association between the status of vitamin D during pregnancy and depression in progenies [30].

Children and Adolescents

Globally depression affects not just adults but also children and adolescents posing a serious health and financial burden [31].

The literature review revealed that increased depressive symptoms were related to inadequate amounts of micronutrients including 25-OHD among children plus adolescents [32].

During pregnancy, a higher concentration of vitamin D in mothers has been linked to better mental health in children [33]. This finding is consistent with other reviewed studies supporting the idea that vitamin D potentially positively influences mental health in children. The results were gathered and organized based on exposure (status of vitamin D supplementation) and outcome (mental health components). The included studies evaluated depressive symptoms and other behavior problems (aggressive disorder, psychotic features, bipolar disorder *etc.*) and general patterns such as the level of distress, quality of life, well-being, mood, and sleep patterns. The studies were conducted in groups of individuals with no mental health issues or in groups of those who had mental health issues. The findings suggested that the intake of vitamin D, either from wholesome diet or through supplementation, besides appropriate sun exposure, should be indicated as an aspect of improving children's psychological well-being. Therefore, it should be advised to achieve the necessary blood level of 25(OH)cholecalciferol for both preventing and treating mental health issues [34].

Cross-sectional research conducted at several governmental high schools in rural India revealed a statistically significant relationship between depression among teenagers and vitamin D levels [35].

A longitudinal study of schoolchildren in Colombia provided insight insight information on the association the associations of deficiency of vitamin D and binding protein for vitamin D in preadolescence with behaviour issues among adolescents. The results of this research suggested that the deficiency of vitamin D in childhood's middle years was positively related to all internalizing and externalizing problems in teenagers. Furthermore, reduced levels of 25-OHD binding protein were linked to increased self-reported aggressive behaviour and symptoms of depressive disorder and anxiousness among schoolchildren [36].

A longitudinal study highlighted a prospective association between baseline vitamin D levels and the risk of depression in early adolescents. Three time periods between 2019 and 2021 were used to evaluate self-reports on depression. Within two-year follow-ups, higher baseline serum levels of 25-OHD were associated with a lower likelihood of cumulative incident depression (adjusted RR = 0.97, 95% CI 0.94-0.99) [37].

Recently, a clinical trial was carried out to investigate the effects of rapid vitamin D_3 supplementation vs untreated vitamin D insufficiency on grades of depression in kids and teenagers. After four weeks of in- or day-patient therapy, the results showed significantly reduced parent-reported symptoms of depression but not self-reported depressive symptoms in comparison with placebo [38].

An observational study on adolescents of middle schools was carried out in Kuwait. Kuwait is a country where deficiency of vitamin D is quite common. The results showed that there was no correlation between symptoms of depression and vitamin D levels. However, for a number of additional health benefits, it is imperative to maintain adequate vitamin D levels throughout adolescence [39].

Adults

Research has been undertaken to look at potential links between depression and vitamin D levels. A recent study in Peshawar examined the serum concentration of vitamin D amongst 100 controls and 100 subjects with depression. The Beck Depression Inventory (BDI) scale was utilised for screening. It was noted that normal subjects had adequate vitamin D levels whereas a slight deficiency was seen in depressed subjects [40]. A systematic review examined a combination of case-control, cross-sectional, and cohort studies to explore the nature of association between vitamin D and depression. Findings revealed that people with depression had lower vitamin D levels. When participants with the lowest and highest serum vitamin D levels were compared, it was observed that those with the lowest levels had elevated odds (OR = 1.31) for depression [41]. Since numerous investigations have observed modest links between depression and vitamin D, experimental studies are being run to further test Vitamin D supplementation in modulating depressive symptoms. A recent review analysed forty-one RCTs published between 2019 to 2022 that tested the effect of vitamin D supplementation in reducing depressive symptoms in adults. The total number of participants included in the meta-analysis was 53,235. Results revealed that adding a vitamin D supplement showed a positive impact on depressive symptoms

(Hedges' g = -0.317, p < 0.001, I2 = 88.16%; GRADE: very low certainty). When the duration of supplementation was altered, *i.e.*, supplementation for fewer than 12 weeks as opposed to more than 12 weeks, the effect of the supplementation seemed to be greater. Furthermore, supplement dosages up to 2,000 IU/day showed a bigger effect than doses up to 4,000 IU daily, with both having small-to-moderate size effects. Also, vitamin D supplementation for the group with vitamin D levels less than 50 nmol/L, falling below the recommended vitamin D level showed slightly better impact. Although the risk of bias assessment was less than ideal in most of the included research papers, the review surmised that supplementing vitamin D at doses of more than 2,000 IU daily seems to lessen symptoms of depression [42]. Some previous studies also observed improvement in the well-being of participants upon the consumption of Vitamin D supplements. For a duration of one to three months, high doses of Vitamin D (more than 100 μg) were supplemented daily, in a group of depressive patients which showed a positive impact on depressive symptoms [43]. It must be noted that reviews and meta-analyses published before that explored causal links between vitamin D supplementation and depression mostly reported mixed findings with weaker indications of possible benefits [41, 44 - 47]. For instance, a review by Gowda *et al.*, analyzed studies carried out on adults who were diagnosed with depressive disorder. No significant improvements in symptoms of depression were observed after Vitamin D supplementation. However, the systematic review by Cheng *et al.* analysed 25 RCTs investigating vitamin D supplementation and its effect on negative emotions. Findings revealed that vitamin D exerted a modest positive effect on negative emotions (Hedges' g = -0.4990, p = .0047, I2 = 97.7%). Furthermore, when supplemented with vitamin D, the subjects with severe depression alongside those whose serum vitamin D was lower than 50 nmol/L, showed modest positive improvements [47]. Pooling the results from vitamin D supplementation trials that lasted longer than 8 weeks with daily dosages exceeding 4,000 IU, demonstrated that vitamin D had a minimal effect [47]. It is worth noting that multiple methodological factors in vitamin D supplementation studies influence the degree of clinical improvement in depressive symptoms. A study that pooled the results of different vitamin D supplementation trials with fewer methodological errors (such as inadequate vitamin D dose) showed greater beneficial effects of vitamin D, whereas trials with methodological errors showed worsening depression symptoms with supplementation [48].

Older Adults

Geriatric depression emerges as the most pervasive mood disorder among the elderly that is linked to higher rates of illness, disability, and death as well as a poorer quality of life. Despite its high prevalence, depression is frequently undiagnosed and poorly treated in this subgroup [49]. This age group is particularly vulnerable to low serum concentrations of vitamin D given their inadequate sunlight exposure coupled with the diminishing production of endogenous vitamin D [50]. A recent community study explored the linkage between incident depression and serum vitamin D in a sample of 4000 healthy participants who were 50 years and older. Baseline results showed that individuals with incident depression were more likely to suffer from low serum vitamin D. Also, individuals with vitamin D deficiency had significantly higher odds of having incident depression (odds ratio 1.75, P = .001). Also, the deficit in vitamin D was linked to a 75% higher chance of developing depression within 4 years. Despite adjusting for significant covariates: physical activity, cardiovascular disease, and use of antidepressants, the aforementioned findings were robustly maintained [51]. Another study analysed six dose-response cohort studies amongst the elderly to delve into the links between depression and serum concentrations of vitamin D. Among 16,287 geriatric participants, 1,157 depressive cases were analysed. The pooled estimate for depression revealed that for each 10 ng per ml increase in Vitamin D concentrations in the blood, the hazard ratio was 0.88 (p <0.001). Vitamin D concentrations and incident depression were found to be correlated linearly in a dose-responsive manner (p = 0.96), indicating that raising vitamin D levels *in vivo* might be a helpful strategy to lower the risk of developing depression among the elderly [52]. Limited research has probed into the effect of Vitamin D supplementation amongst older adults concerning depressive symptoms. In the review published recently on Vitamin D supplementation and depression, the authors observed that the supplementation of vitamin D failed to confer any significant impact on depressive symptoms in the trials conducted amongst the elderly (more than 65 years) thus limiting generalizability [42]. This review included two studies investigating this relationship in older adults. The first study, the D-Vitaal study investigated the impact of vitamin D supplementation on depressive symptomatology in 155 participants who ranged from 60 to 80 years with low vitamin D status. The intervention group was supplemented with 1200 IU of vitamin D per day for 12 months. Subsequently, a modest improvement in concentrations of serum vitamin D concentrations was noted in the intervention group. However, no benefit was seen in elderly patients with low serum concentrations of vitamin D [53]. The second trial for vitamin D supplementation was an RCT that lasted for 8 weeks. 78 older adults (60 years and older), with moderate to severe levels of depression were allotted to be part of either the experimental or placebo group in a random fashion. The experimental group was given 50,000 IU of vitamin D_3 weekly for 8 weeks. This group, which previously had a depression score of 9.25 experienced a significant drop in the depression score to 7.48 (p = 0.0001), suggesting that vitamin D supplements may help in symptom reduction in the elderly with depression. However, the small sample size of the population limits generalizability [54]. It is worth adding that the appropriate dosages for vitamin D may be different for the elderly. This difference could be attributed to physiological and neurobiological changes that are known to accompany aging processes [42, 55]. Thus, more extensive clinical studies should be carried out to examine the possible advantages of vitamin D in reducing symptoms of depression amongst this vulnerable subset of the population.

CONCLUSION

The scientific evidence is strongly supportive of a connection between depression and vitamin D. However, numerous discrepancies remain, and further investigations must address the limitations. To improve our understanding and therapeutic strategy, more well-designed trials are required that utilize standard tests, dosing regimens and indicators of outcome.

REFERENCES

[1]   Saponaro F, Saba A, Zucchi RJIjoms. An update on vitamin D metabolism. 2020; 21(18): 6573.

[2]   Al-Zohily B, Al-Menhali A, Gariballa S, Haq A. Shah IJIjoms. Epimers of vitamin D: a review. 2020; 21(2): 470.

[3]   Khammissa R, Fourie J, Motswaledi M, Ballyram R, Lemmer J, Feller LJBri. The biological activities of vitamin D and its receptor in relation to calcium and bone homeostasis, cancer, immune and cardiovascular systems, skin biology, and oral health. 2018; 2018.

[4]   Haussler MR, Whitfield GK, Kaneko I, *et al.* Molecular mechanisms of vitamin D action. 2013; 92: 77-98.
        [http://dx.doi.org/10.1007/s00223-012-9619-0]

[5]   Cui A, Zhang T, Xiao P, Fan Z, Wang H, Zhuang Y. Global and regional prevalence of vitamin D deficiency in population-based studies from 2000 to 2022: A pooled analysis of 7.9 million participants. Front Nutr 2023; 10: 1070808.
        [http://dx.doi.org/10.3389/fnut.2023.1070808] [PMID: 37006940]

[6]   Santos HO, Martins CEC, Forbes SC, Delpino FM. A scoping review of vitamin D for nonskeletal health: A framework for evidence-based clinical practice. Clin Ther 2023; 45(5): e127-50.
        [http://dx.doi.org/10.1016/j.clinthera.2023.03.016] [PMID: 37080887]

[7]   World Health Organization W. Depressive disorder (depression) fact sheet 2023 [Available from: https://www.who.int/news-room/fact-sheets/detail/depression#:~:text=Depressive%20disorder%20

[8]   Ljungberg T, Bondza E, Lethin C. Evidence of the importance of dietary habits regarding depressive symptoms and depression 2020; 17(5): 1616.

[9]   Xiong P, Liu M, Liu B, Hall BJ. Trends in the incidence and DALYs of anxiety disorders at the global, regional, and national levels: Estimates from the Global Burden of Disease Study 2019. J Affect Disord 2022; 297: 83-93.
        [http://dx.doi.org/10.1016/j.jad.2021.10.022] [PMID: 34678404]

[10]   Owen L, Corfe B. The role of diet and nutrition on mental health and wellbeing. Proc Nutr Soc 2017; 76(4): 425-6.
        [http://dx.doi.org/10.1017/S0029665117001057] [PMID: 28707609]

[11]   Kouba BR, Camargo A, Gil-Mohapel J, Rodrigues ALS. Molecular basis underlying the therapeutic

potential of vitamin D for the treatment of depression and anxiety. 2022; 23(13): 7077.
[http://dx.doi.org/10.3390/ijms23137077]

[12] Beurel E, Toups M, Nemeroff CBJN. The bidirectional relationship of depression and inflammation: double trouble. 2020; 107(2): 234-56.
[http://dx.doi.org/10.1016/j.neuron.2020.06.002]

[13] Tang M, Liu T, Jiang P, Dang RJPr. The interaction between autophagy and neuroinflammation in major depressive disorder: from pathophysiology to therapeutic implications. 2021; 168: 105586.

[14] Casseb GA, Kaster MP, Rodrigues ALSJCd. Potential role of vitamin D for the management of depression and anxiety. 2019; 33(7): 619-37.

[15] Berridge MJJPr. Vitamin D and depression: cellular and regulatory mechanisms. 2017; 69(2): 80-92.

[16] Menon V, Kar SK, Suthar N, Nebhinani NJIjopm. Vitamin D and depression: a critical appraisal of the evidence and future directions. 2020; 42(1): 11-21.

[17] Brigitta BJDicn. Pathophysiology of depression and mechanisms of treatment. 2022.

[18] Bian Q, Wang J, editors. Tryptophan hydroxylase 2 and tryptophan mediate depression by regulating serotonin levels. AIP Conference Proceedings; 2022: AIP Publishing.
[http://dx.doi.org/10.1063/5.0096466]

[19] Geng C, Shaikh AS, Han W, Chen D, Guo Y, Jiang P. Vitamin D and depression: mechanisms, determination and application. Asia Pac J Clin Nutr 2019; 28(4): 689-94.
[PMID: 31826364]

[20] Lisakovska O, Labudzynskyi D, Khomenko A, *et al.* Brain vitamin D3-auto/paracrine system in relation to structural, neurophysiological, and behavioral disturbances associated with glucocorticoid-induced neurotoxicity. 2023; 17: 1133400.

[21] Gáll Z, Székely OJN. Role of vitamin D in cognitive dysfunction: New molecular concepts and discrepancies between animal and human findings. 2021; 13(11): 3672.

[22] Shi Y, Song R, Wang L, *et al.* Identifying Plasma Biomarkers with high specificity for major depressive disorder: A multi-level proteomics study. J Affect Disord 2020; 277: 620-30.
[http://dx.doi.org/10.1016/j.jad.2020.08.078] [PMID: 32905914]

[23] Parel NS, Krishna PV, Gupta A, *et al.* Depression and vitamin D: a peculiar relationship. 2022; 14(4).

[24] Stoica AB, Mărginean C. The impact of vitamin D deficiency on infants' health. Nutrients 2023; 15(20): 4379.
[http://dx.doi.org/10.3390/nu15204379] [PMID: 37892454]

[25] Mo H, Zhang J, Huo C, *et al.* The association of vitamin D deficiency, age and depression in US adults: a cross-sectional analysis. 2023; 23(1): 534.
[http://dx.doi.org/10.1186/s12888-023-04685-0]

[26] Lisi G, Ribolsi M, Siracusano A, Niolu C. Maternal vitamin D and its role in determining fetal origins of mental health. Curr Pharm Des 2020; 26(21): 2497-509.
[http://dx.doi.org/10.2174/1381612826666200506093858] [PMID: 32370709]

[27] Ideraabdullah FY, Belenchia AM, Rosenfeld CS, *et al.* Maternal vitamin D deficiency and developmental origins of health and disease (DOHaD). J Endocrinol 2019; 241(2): R65-80.
[http://dx.doi.org/10.1530/JOE-18-0541] [PMID: 30909167]

[28] Arshad R, Sameen A, Murtaza MA, *et al.* Impact of vitamin D on maternal and fetal health: A review. Food Sci Nutr 2022; 10(10): 3230-40.
[http://dx.doi.org/10.1002/fsn3.2948] [PMID: 36249984]

[29] Strøm M, Halldorsson TI, Hansen S, *et al.* Vitamin D measured in maternal serum and offspring neurodevelopmental outcomes: a prospective study with long-term follow-up. Ann Nutr Metab 2014; 64(3-4): 254-61.

[http://dx.doi.org/10.1159/000365030] [PMID: 25300268]

[30]   Wang MJ, Dunn EC, Okereke OI, Kraft P, Zhu Y, Smoller JW. Maternal vitamin D status during pregnancy and offspring risk of childhood/adolescent depression: Results from the Avon Longitudinal Study of Parents and Children (ALSPAC). J Affect Disord 2020; 265: 255-62.
[http://dx.doi.org/10.1016/j.jad.2020.01.005] [PMID: 32090749]

[31]   Föcker M, Antel J, Grasemann C, *et al.* Effect of an vitamin D deficiency on depressive symptoms in child and adolescent psychiatric patients – a randomized controlled trial: study protocol. BMC Psychiatry 2018; 18(1): 57.
[http://dx.doi.org/10.1186/s12888-018-1637-7] [PMID: 29490621]

[32]   Campisi SC, Zasowski C, Shah S, *et al.* Assessing the evidence of micronutrients on depression among children and adolescents: An evidence gap map. Adv Nutr 2020; 11(4): 908-27.
[http://dx.doi.org/10.1093/advances/nmaa021] [PMID: 32193537]

[33]   Sammallahti S, Holmlund-Suila E, Zou R, *et al.* Prenatal maternal and cord blood vitamin D concentrations and negative affectivity in infancy. Eur Child Adolesc Psychiatry 2023; 32(4): 601-9.
[http://dx.doi.org/10.1007/s00787-021-01894-4] [PMID: 34657965]

[34]   Głąbska D, Kołota A, Lachowicz K, Skolmowska D, Stachoń M, Guzek D. The influence of vitamin D intake and status on mental health in children: A systematic review. Nutrients 2021; 13(3): 952.
[http://dx.doi.org/10.3390/nu13030952] [PMID: 33809478]

[35]   Satyanarayana PT, Suryanarayana R, Yesupatham ST, Reddy S, Reddy N, Pradeep TJC. Is sunshine vitamin related to adolescent depression? a cross-sectional study of vitamin D status and depression among rural adolescents. 2023; 15(2).

[36]   Robinson SL, Marín C, Oliveros H, *et al.* Vitamin D deficiency in middle childhood is related to behavior problems in adolescence. J Nutr 2020; 150(1): 140-8.
[http://dx.doi.org/10.1093/jn/nxz185] [PMID: 31429909]

[37]   Wang G, Yuan M, Chang J, Li Y, Blum R, Su P. Vitamin D and depressive symptoms in an early adolescent cohort. Psychol Med 2023; 53(12): 5852-60.
[http://dx.doi.org/10.1017/S0033291722003117] [PMID: 37795689]

[38]   Libuda L, Timmesfeld N, Antel J, *et al.* Effect of vitamin D deficiency on depressive symptoms in child and adolescent psychiatric patients: results of a randomized controlled trial. Eur J Nutr 2020; 59(8): 3415-24.
[http://dx.doi.org/10.1007/s00394-020-02176-6] [PMID: 32108263]

[39]   Al-Sabah R, Al-Taiar A, Shaban L, Albatineh AN, Sharaf Alddin R, Durgampudi PK. Vitamin D level in relation to depression symptoms during adolescence. Child Adolesc Psychiatry Ment Health 2022; 16(1): 53.
[http://dx.doi.org/10.1186/s13034-022-00489-4] [PMID: 35761369]

[40]   Khan B, Shafiq H, Abbas S, Jabeen S, *et al.* Vitamin D status and its correlation to depression. Annals of General Psychiatry. 2022; 21(1): 32.

[41]   Anglin RES, Samaan Z, Walter SD, McDonald SD. Vitamin D deficiency and depression in adults: systematic review and meta-analysis. Br J Psychiatry 2013; 202(2): 100-7.
[http://dx.doi.org/10.1192/bjp.bp.111.106666] [PMID: 23377209]

[42]   Mikola T, Marx W, Lane MM, *et al.* The effect of vitamin D supplementation on depressive symptoms in adults: A systematic review and meta-analysis of randomized controlled trials. Crit Rev Food Sci Nutr 2022; 1-18.
[PMID: 35816192]

[43]   Li G, Mbuagbaw L, Samaan Z, *et al.* Efficacy of vitamin D supplementation in depression in adults: a systematic review protocol. Syst Rev 2013; 2(1): 64.
[http://dx.doi.org/10.1186/2046-4053-2-64] [PMID: 23927040]

[44]   Li G, Mbuagbaw L, Samaan Z, *et al.* Efficacy of vitamin D supplementation in depression in adults: a

systematic review. J Clin Endocrinol Metab 2014; 99(3): 757-67.
[http://dx.doi.org/10.1210/jc.2013-3450] [PMID: 24423304]

[45]   Gowda U, Mutowo MP, Smith BJ, Wluka AE, Renzaho AMN. Vitamin D supplementation to reduce depression in adults: Meta-analysis of randomized controlled trials. Nutrition 2015; 31(3): 421-9.
[http://dx.doi.org/10.1016/j.nut.2014.06.017] [PMID: 25701329]

[46]   Vellekkatt F, Menon V. Efficacy of vitamin D supplementation in major depression. J Postgrad Med 2019; 65(2): 74-80.
[http://dx.doi.org/10.4103/jpgm.JPGM_571_17] [PMID: 29943744]

[47]   Cheng Y-C, Huang Y-C, Huang W-L. The effect of vitamin D supplement on negative emotions: A systematic review and meta-analysis. 2020; 37(6): 549-64.
[http://dx.doi.org/10.1002/da.23025]

[48]   Spedding S. Vitamin D and depression: A systematic review and meta-analysis comparing studies with and without biological flaws. 2014; 6(4): 1501-18.
[http://dx.doi.org/10.3390/nu6041501]

[49]   Devita M, De Salvo R, Ravelli A, *et al.* Recognizing depression in the elderly: practical guidance and challenges for clinical management. Neuropsychiatric Disease and Treatment. 2022; 18: 2867-80.

[50]   Amrein K, Scherkl M, Hoffmann M, *et al.* Vitamin D deficiency 2.0: an update on the current status worldwide. Eur J Clin Nutr 2020; 74(11): 1498-513.
[http://dx.doi.org/10.1038/s41430-020-0558-y] [PMID: 31959942]

[51]   Briggs R, McCarroll K, O'Halloran A, *et al.* Vitamin D deficiency is associated with an increased likelihood of incident depression in community-dwelling older adults. J Am Med Dir Assoc 2019; 20(5): 517-23.
[http://dx.doi.org/10.1016/j.jamda.2018.10.006] [PMID: 30470577]

[52]   Li H, Sun D, Wang A, *et al.* Serum 25-hydroxyvitamin d levels and depression in older adults: A dose–response meta-analysis of prospective cohort studies. Am J Geriatr Psychiatry 2019; 27(11): 1192-202.
[http://dx.doi.org/10.1016/j.jagp.2019.05.022] [PMID: 31262683]

[53]   De Koning EJ, Lips P, Penninx BWJH, *et al.* Vitamin D supplementation for the prevention of depression and poor physical function in older persons: the D-Vitaal study, a randomized clinical trial. Am J Clin Nutr 2019; 110(5): 1119-30.
[http://dx.doi.org/10.1093/ajcn/nqz141] [PMID: 31340012]

[54]   Alavi NM, Khademalhoseini S, Vakili Z, Assarian F. Effect of vitamin D supplementation on depression in elderly patients: A randomized clinical trial. Clin Nutr 2019; 38(5): 2065-70.
[http://dx.doi.org/10.1016/j.clnu.2018.09.011] [PMID: 30316534]

[55]   Okereke OI, Singh A. The role of vitamin D in the prevention of late-life depression. J Affect Disord 2016; 198: 1-14.
[http://dx.doi.org/10.1016/j.jad.2016.03.022] [PMID: 26998791]

CHAPTER 7

Vitamin D and Melanoma

Shaikha Alnaqbi[1,*], **Noor Abu Dheir**[1] and **Dimitrios Papandreou**[1]

[1] *Department of Clinical Nutrition and Dietetics, College of Health Sciences, University of Sharjah, Sharjah, UAE*

Abstract: Melanoma, a malignant tumor of the skin, is a major health concern worldwide, with increased incidence rates especially among fair-skinned individuals. This section investigates the complex connection between vitamin D and melanoma, offering insight to vitamin D's numerous functions in both skin health and prevention of cancer. Vitamin D, which is largely synthesized in the skin in response to ultraviolet B (UVB) radiation, has important activities beyond mineral homeostasis, such as immunological regulation and tumor suppression. Considering its potential preventive effects, the processes behind vitamin D's influence on the likelihood of melanoma and progression are complex and require further research. Observational studies indicate a possible adverse link between vitamin D levels and melanoma risk, while causality and appropriate supplementing regimens are unclear. Genetic differences in vitamin D receptors and metabolic enzymes may also influence an individual's vulnerability to melanoma. Melanoma risk reduction strategies include a broad approach, including limiting UV exposure, supplementing the diet, and considering genetics. This review summarizes the current investigation into vitamin D's complex interaction with melanoma, emphasizing the necessity for comprehensive measures to maximize its efficacy in melanoma prevention and care.

Keywords: Melanoma, Risk factor, Sunlight exposure, Vitamin D, 25-Hydroxyvitamin D.

INTRODUCTION

Malignant melanoma arises from the dermis, a layer of the skin. Despite being the third most common skin cancer, it is the primary cause of melanoma-related deaths and its incidence is increasing [1]. Its incidence is strongly connected with skin color and geographic area. Outdoor activity modifications and solar exposure over the last seventy years are significant contributors to the rising incidence of melanoma [2].

* **Corresponding author Shaikha Alnaqbi:** Department of Clinical Nutrition and Dietetics, College of Health Sciences, University of Sharjah, Sharjah, UAE; E-mails: U23102372@sharjah.ac.ae, shaikhaealnaqbi@gmail.com

Melanoma

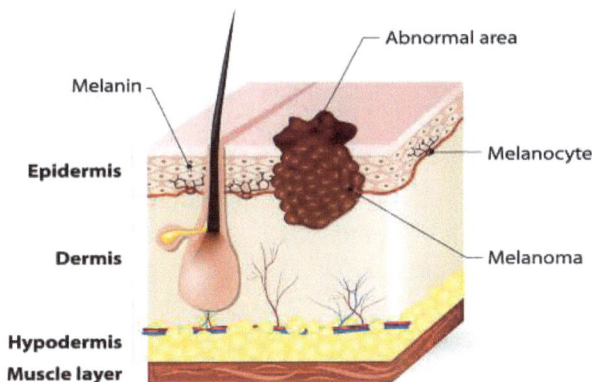

Melanoma is responsible for 1.7% of cancer occurrences worldwide and is the fifth most prominent malignancy in the United States. Melanoma in developed, fair-skinned nations has increased by over 320% in the United States. Since 2011, ten new targeted or immunotherapy agents have been approved in the United States, leading to a decrease in the mortality of nearly 30% over the past decade [3]. The different types of cancers are described below in Table **1**. [4]

Table 1. Different types of cancer and fatalities.

Rank	Typical Forms of Cancer	New Instances in 2023	Approximate Fatalities in 2023
1.	Breast Cancer Female	297,790	43,170
2.	Prostate Cancer	288,300	34,700
3.	Lung and Bronchus Cancer	238,340	127,070
4.	Colorectal Cancer	153,020	52,550
5.	**Melanoma of the Skin**	**97,610**	**7,990**
6.	Bladder Cancer	82,290	16,710
7.	Kidney and Renal Pelvis Cancer	81,800	14,890
8.	Non-Hodgkin Lymphoma	80,550	20,180
9.	Uterine Cancer	66,200	13,030

Cancer Facts Sheets, 2023 [4].

The existing treatments encompass a range of interventions such as chemotherapy, photodynamic treatment, immunotherapy, surgical interventions, and targeted therapy are all options. The treatment approach can consist of the utilization of either individual drugs or a combination of therapies, based on factors such as the patient's overall well, tumor location and stage. The effectiveness of these interventions may be diminished because of the emergence of various resistance mechanisms [5].

Approximately 90% of vitamin D is produced in the skin when exposed to the sun, predominantly the ultraviolet type B (UVB) spectrum [6].

Vitamin D is actually a genuine hormone that the human body can produce when exposed to sunlight or through a well-rounded and nutritious diet that includes vitamin D-rich foods or supplements. Unfortunately, our prevalent indoor lifestyle, coupled with irregular and insufficient exposure to sunlight, as well as various factors like human migration, has led to a widespread deficiency of vitamin D. Ironically, this deficiency is occurring simultaneously with a rise in the prevalence of skin cancer in certain regions [7].

Maintaining a healthy level of vitamin D is essential for strong bones. D hypovitaminosis disorders, such as rickets, and osteomalacia, have been well described and should be prevented whenever possible. However, D hypovitaminosis may also be implicated in loss of bone mass, sarcopenia, falls, as well as frailty fractures in the elderly, which are major public health concerns in Europe due to their impact on morbidity, quality of life, and the cost of healthcare [8].

Vitamin D is popular for its involvement in mineral homeostasis regulation; nevertheless, D hypovitaminosis has also been related to the development and progression of certain cancer types [9].

When the skin is placed under the sun, UV B photons penetrate it and break down 7-dehydrocholesterol into pre-vitamin D3. This pre-vitamin D3 is then transformed into vitamin D3 through a process called isomerization, which is facilitated by the body's temperature. The majority of mankind have relied on the sun to meet their vitamin D needs. Factors such as skin pigmentation, sunscreen application, aging, time of day, season, and latitude have a significant impact on the synthesis of previtamin D3 [10].

Due to its high incidence and mortality rate, melanoma is a major clinical issue that affects many people. UVR, or ultraviolet light, is a major contributor to the carcinogenic alteration of melanocytes and the development of melanoma. However, UVB is needed for the cutaneous generation of vitamin D3, despite its role as a complete carcinogen in melanoma genesis [11].

In a study of 87 patients with malignant melanoma to investigate the impact that vitamin D may have on the outcome of patients with melanoma, only 11 patients

(12.7%) displayed normal levels of vitamin D in their blood irrespective of the anatomical site of the melanoma. Hence, the amounts of vitamin D are thought to help protect against melanoma. Many observational research studies have been conducted to compare the amounts of vitamin D to the outcomes of malignant melanoma. Slominski *et al.* suggest increasing the amount of vitamin D consumption by 10,000 IU per day or 50,000 IU every week for people with stage 3 or 4 melanoma. More research is needed to determine the processes underlying the relationship between vitamin D and cancerous melanoma. More research would be needed to determine whether people with melanoma should be recommended to take supplements of vitamin D or just increase their exposure to the sun [12].

UV Light Exposure, Protection and Sun Avoidance

Vitamin D delivers its effects *via* its contact with the nuclear vitamin D receptor. These are found in all human tissues. Calcitriol stimulates differentiation and movement into the outer layer of the skin while inhibiting keratinocyte and melanocyte growth *in vitro via* the vitamin D receptor inside the epidermis [13].

Vitamin D receptor functions as a tumor suppressor, and its production has been associated to the rapid growth of cancerous melanoma [14]. According to growing evidence, a combination of oncogenic installation, increased metabolic rate, and mitochondrial malfunction appears to worsen underlying reactive oxygen species stress in tumor cells. It is well known that the respiratory pathway of mitochondria generates reactive oxygen species in cells. Tumor cells may be subjected to reactive oxygen species stress in one form since their DNA is sensitive to reactive oxygen species damage. As a result, mitochondria have been related to the development of cancer [15] as an outcome of their roles as reactive oxygen species makers and participants in programmed cell death and other aspects of tumor physiology [16].

It has been suggested that the build-up of mutations in mitochondrial DNA (mtDNA) is a fundamental factor in the aging process, and these mutations have been linked to cancer in various tissues, including the skin of humans [17].

Among the multiple variables contributing to the development of melanoma, such as genetic susceptibility, immune system suppression, and exposure to UV radiation, reducing UV exposure has garnered the greatest focus in efforts to mitigate the public health impact of melanoma [18].

Indoor tanning beds elevate the likelihood of developing melanoma and nonmelanoma skin cancer. Indoor tanning beds have emerged as significant contributors to UVB and UVA ultraviolet (UV) exposure [19].

The timing of when women began indoor tanning in relation to their diagnosis suggests that indoor tanning is a probable contributing cause to the higher increase in melanoma rates among younger women compared to males in the United States. Unless there are restrictions and reductions on indoor tanning, the melanoma epidemic is likely to persist [20].

The utilization of tanning booths can lead to elevated levels of serum vitamin D. However, this effect may be complicated by the longer total period of sun exposure among individuals who utilize tanning booths [21].

Skin color may also affect the risk of melanoma. Multiple researches examined the relationship between UV exposure and the liklihood of cutaneous melanoma in individuals with dark skin of color. The evidence indicates that UV exposure may not significantly contribute to the development of melanoma in those with darker skin tones. Recent evidence also does not support the current recommendations that advocate for UV protection in order to prevent melanoma in individuals with darker skin tones [22].

While sun avoidance is considered crucial in mitigating the impact of melanocytic and keratinocytic malignancies on public health, efforts to promote sun avoidance through educational and media campaigns have not successfully resulted in the desired behavioral modifications among young individuals. Additionally, these campaigns had a limited effect on elderly patients who have already endured years of harmful sun exposure. Most significantly, these initiatives have not succeeded in reducing the occurrence of melanoma [18].

The possibility of extra endogenous photoprotection by dietary antioxidants has also generated significant interest. Several effective micronutrients can help reduce the damage caused by UV in humans. These compounds protect specific molecular sites by neutralizing harmful reactive oxygen species, including excited singlet oxygen and molecules in a triplet state. Additionally, they manage signaling pathways activated by stress and/or impede cellular and tissue reactions, including inflammation. The existence of micronutrients within diet, like carotenoids, vitamins E and C, and polyphenols, supports the body's antioxidant defenses and may additionally play a role in the innate shielding mechanisms against sunlight [23].

It has been found in several cohort studies that caffeine has a protective effect against skin cancer, thus being the most promising substance in this field. Regardless of solid evidence from cellular and animal experiments, the practical significance of vitamin D and zinc's immune-modulating characteristics, polyphenols' anti-angiogenic possibilities, and flavonoids' cell growth-inhibiting impact has been extremely limited in healthcare settings due to a lack of human research [24].

Vitamin D Derivatives and Melanoma

We know that Calcitriol is the vitamin D's initial active form. It primarily functions *via* attaching to the VDR (Vitamin D Receptor) nuclear. When calcitriol activates VDR, it forms a complex with the retinoid X receptor (RXR), moves into the cell nucleus, and attaches to the VDR-responding element to function as a transcription factor.

Depending on the kind of cell, there are more than 1,000 target genes that are substantially varied in their biological activity and controlled by vitamin D.

Many tissues and cells, including epidermal and dermal skin cells that both produce and react to Calcitriol, have been shown to express VDR. VDR can also be influenced by other hydroxylated vitamin D shapes that are non-standard and non-calcemic.

Additionally, they can function as contrary agonists on RORs (retinoic acid-related orphan receptors) α and γ, which are expressed in healthy and diseased dermis cells, as well as melanoma. The capacity of vitamin D3 hydroxy-derivatives to interact with the aryl hydrocarbon receptor has most recently been demonstrated. The many functions of vitamin D might be connected to different vitamin D3 receptors and metabolites. Promising options for the avoidance and therapy of melanoma include vitamin D and its latest compounds (Fig. **1**) [25].

Research evidence has shown that raised measures of vitamin D are associated with a lessened likelihood of melanoma development and recurrence [26] though it's not certain if vitamin D provides protection on its own or serves as a stand-in for other protective elements [27].

Additionally, it was suggested that higher vitamin D measures correlate with healthier lifestyles, which offer overall cancer prevention [28, 29].

Potential Role of Vitamin D in Melanoma

Latest data indicates that vitamin D possesses immune-modulating characteristics that have been extensively studied in autoimmune disorders, as well as anti-proliferative actions on tumour cells [27]. The cancer-fighting capabilities of vitamin D have sparked a growing interest in oncology during the last few years. Most patients with melanoma have D hypovitaminosis for a variety of reasons, such as malnourishment and insufficient sun exposure. During anti-cancer therapy, there is a chance of both unfavourable skin events and skin cancers that progress over time [30]. Furthermore, melanoma thickness and poor survival have been linked to vitamin D hypovitaminosis lending support to the theory that vitamin D derivatives may be crucial in the avoidance and therapy of cancer [31].

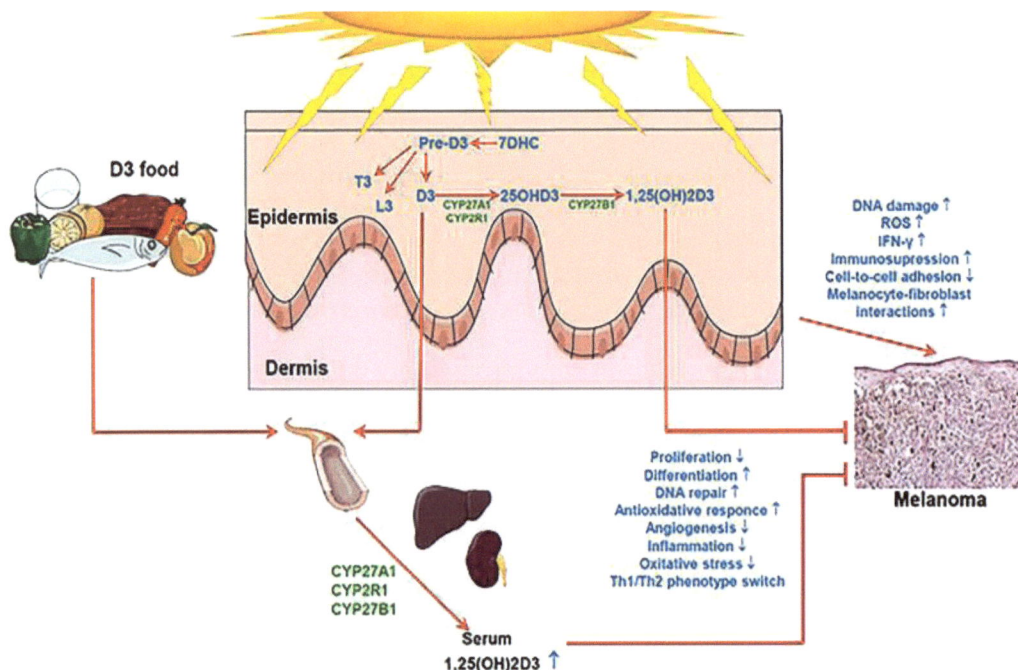

Fig. (1). Diagram showing vitamin D production, activation, and its implications over melanoma biology. **Adapted with permission from** [25].

In fact, high-risk melanoma patients who received adjuvant vitamin D3 (cholecalciferol) have achieved enhancements in both survival without progression and overall survival [32]. This suggests that the treatment may be beneficial. Despite its anti-cancer characteristics, vitamin D has been also shown to have immunosuppressive properties, therefore this therapy method is still not regarded as the "standard of care."

In fact, there is evidence that vitamin D can elevate the ratio of T-regulatory to T-helper 17 cells in the tumour microenvironment, leading to immunological suppression [33]

Exploring The Link Between Vitamin D and Non-Melanoma Skin Cancer

This study carried out a systematic review of the literature to look into the possible link between non-melanoma skin cancer (NMSC) risk and vitamin D levels in the blood, vitamin D intake from food or dietary supplements, or particular genetic variants at the VDR or VDBP genes [34] (Table **2**).

Table 2. Relation of Vitamin D and Non-Melanoma Skin Cancer.

Correlation Studies	Number of Studies	Main Results
Vitamin D levels in The Blood and The Risk of NMSC	10 Studies	-Two patient-based research that indicated no link between serum vitamin D levels and Squamous Cell Carcinoma risk were omitted from the meta-analysis of 1192 kidney transplant recipients. One study indicated that D hypovitaminosis increased the probability of Basal Cell Carcinoma with an Odds Ratio of 2.62 and 95% CI 2.42–2.85 and Squamous Cell Carcinoma with an Odds Ratio of 2.89 and 95% CI 2.61–3.20 in patients with Crohn's disease. - Three of the six investigations discovered a dose-response association between vitamin D levels and the risk of NMSC. -The random effects meta-analysis found a 67% increase in non-melanoma skin cancer (NMSC) risk among individuals with the maximum vitamin D levels in comparison to those with the lowest levels. However, this increase was not statistically significant, with a confidence interval of 0.61-4.56.
NMSC Risk and Vitamin D From Both Food Intake and Dietary Supplements	5 Studies	-There is no notable correlation between the consumption of dietary vitamin D and the risk of developing basal cell carcinoma (BCC). - The population-specific case-control study found no statistically significant association. - Individuals who consume the greatest percentile of total vitamin D intake from food and supplements are more likely to develop BCC, but not SCC. -Two randomized controlled trials (RCTs), both done in the United States, looked into the possibility of non-melanoma skin cancer between those who received vitamin D supplementation and those who received placebo in the control group. However, no significant link was found.
NMSC Risk and VDR (Apa1, Bsm1, Cdx2, Fok1, and Taq1), VDBP Genes Variations.	5 Studies	- Using either the Hom vs. WT or Het vs. WT models, no connection with NMSC risk was found for any of the three genes investigated in the meta-analysis (Apa1, Bsm1, and Taq1). -All models have heterogeneity percentages < 50%. - There was no significant link between Cdx2 or Fok1 gene and NMSC chance in any of the fitted models. - The Fok1 TT (Hom) gene was observed to significantly enhance BCC likelihood with Odds Ratio of 10.14 and p-value of 0.001.
NMSC Risk and The VDBP Gene Variants	1 Study	Despite some evidence of an age-related effect, neither of the two VDBP polymorphisms (rs7041 nor rs4588) studied were linked to BCC.

Caini *et al.* 2021 [34].

Vitamin D Receptor Genetic Variations with the Onset of Cutaneous Melanoma

It has been shown that Vitamin D suppresses adaptive immunity while increasing natural immunity. Eleven new cohort studies investigated the relationship between vitamin D levels and the likelihood of melanoma and prognosis. The correlations found in this research did not have consistent strengths or levels of statistical significance. A systematic review and meta-analysis of research was carried on to assess the effects of high levels of 25(OH)D, the body's main shape of vitamin D, on the onset and progress of melanoma [35] (Table **3**).

Table 3. Correlation studies of vitamin D and Melanoma.

Correlation Studies	Number of Studies	Main Results
The Relationship Between Food Consumption of Vitamin D Serum Levels and The Likelihood of Melanoma	6 Studies	- The data indicate that there is no significant relationship between vitamin D use and blood levels of 25(OH) D with the likelihood of melanoma.
The Relationship Between Levels of Vitamin D in The Blood and The Likelihood of Melanoma	6 Studies	- However, we did find a negative connection between 25(OH)D levels in the blood and the thickness of melanoma, which was recognized as a predictive indicator.
The Relationship Between Vitamin D Levels in Blood and Breslow Thickness	4 Studies	Three of these studies found a negative relationship between levels of 25(OH)D in the blood and the thickness of melanoma.

Song *et al.* 2022 [35].

The study's findings revealed that there was no clear link between vitamin D usage and blood levels of 25(OH)D with the likelihood of melanoma. However, a negative connection was discovered between 25(OH)D concentrations in the blood and the thickness of melanoma. Given the established positive relationship between melanoma thickness and the likelihood of death from melanoma, it is reasonable to conclude that providing melanoma patients with a moderate dietary supplement of vitamin D in order to prevent a deficiency in serum levels may improve their long-term survival [35].

Melanoma and Breslow Thickness

Breslow thickness, which measures the microscopic extent between the epidermis's top layer and the deepest point of cancer dissemination, as well as the occurrence of ulceration are the strongest indicators of survival from melanoma. In patients with thin melanomas, the level of occupation (Clark level) is a powerful predictor (1 mm or less) [36].

The stage of melanoma significantly affects survival rates; 10-year life span ranges from 93% for the thinnest malignancy showing no signs of progression to 39% for large malignancy, showing signs of progression [37].

Vitamin D Levels in Melanoma and Breslow Thickness

Comparing individuals with thinner tumours to those with larger, or higher-stage, melanomas reveals that the latter have a lower vitamin D level. While the results of experimental research have been inconsistent, some indicate that administering vitamin D metabolites may lessen the aggressiveness of tumours. A study examined the association between D hypovitaminosis in patients diagnosed with Melanoma and the Breslow thickness and found that the posibility of having a thicker tumour was approximately four times higher when vitamin D3 was less than 50 nmol/L as the odds ratio was found to be equal to 3.82, with a 95% CI: 1.03, 14.14 and p-value of 0.04, adjusted for age, sex, skin type, BMI, and season of diagnosis). A lower survival is linked to thicker tumours, which are related to alleviated vitamin D measures at the time of melanoma detection. Total 18% of melanomas in this population may have Breslow thicknesses of less than 0.75 mm instead of more than 0.75 mm if vitamin D levels are maintained at 50 nmol/L or above [38].

It is suggested to always maintain vitamin D measures of ≥50 nmol/L as the findings revealed that bigger melanomas, which have been separately shown to have an unfavourable outcome, are linked to D hypovitaminosis. The advantages of sun exposure for achieving "sufficiency" in vitamin D must be balanced in opposition to the potential chances of developing melanoma [39].

CONCLUSION

Finally, studies have found a link between higher vitamin D levels and a lower risk of melanoma. Serum vitamin D levels were discovered to have an inverse connection with the thickness of melanoma, making it a predictive indication. Vitamin D therapy is not yet the "standard of care" due to immune-suppressive side effects, emphasising the significance of combining the benefits of vitamin D with the risks of skin tumours.

REFERENCES

[1]   Davey MG, Miller N, McInerney NM, Davey MG, Miller N, McInerney NM. A review of epidemiology and cancer biology of malignant melanoma. Cureus 2021; 13(5): e15087.
       [http://dx.doi.org/10.7759/cureus.15087] [PMID: 34155457]

[2]   Leiter U, Keim U, Garbe C. Epidemiology of skin cancer: Update 2019. Adv Exp Med Biol 2020; 1268: 123-39.
       [http://dx.doi.org/10.1007/978-3-030-46227-7_6] [PMID: 32918216]

[3]   Saginala K, Barsouk A, Aluru JS, Rawla P, Barsouk A. Epidemiology of Melanoma. Medical Sciences. 2021; 9(4).
[http://dx.doi.org/10.3390/medsci9040063]

[4]   Available from: https://seer.cancer.gov/statfacts/ html/melan.html

[5]   Domingues B, Lopes JM, Soares P, Pópulo H. Melanoma treatment in review. Immunotargets Ther. 2018;7:35.
[http://dx.doi.org/10.2147/ITT.S134842]

[6]   Martin-Gorgojo A, Gilaberte Y, Nagore E. Vitamin D and Skin Cancer: An epidemiological, patient-centered update and review. Nutrients. 2021; 13(12).

[7]   Gilaberte Y, Aguilera J, Carrascosa JM, Figueroa FL, Romaní de Gabriel J, Nagore E. La vitamina D: evidencias y controversias. Actas Dermo-Sifiliográficas (English Edition) 2011; 102(8): 572-88.
[http://dx.doi.org/10.1016/j.adengl.2011.03.013] [PMID: 21620350]

[8]   Spiro A, Buttriss JL, Vitamin D. Vitamin D : An overview of vitamin D status and intake in E urope. Nutr Bull 2014; 39(4): 322-50.
[http://dx.doi.org/10.1111/nbu.12108] [PMID: 25635171]

[9]   Seraphin G, Rieger S, Hewison M, Capobianco E, Lisse TS. The impact of vitamin D on cancer: A mini review. J Steroid Biochem Mol Biol 2023; 231: 106308.
[http://dx.doi.org/10.1016/j.jsbmb.2023.106308] [PMID: 37054849]

[10]   Holick MF. Sunlight, ultraviolet radiation, vitamin D and skin cancer. sunlight, vitamin D and skin cancer. 2014; 1–16.
[http://dx.doi.org/10.1007/978-1-4939-0437-2_1]

[11]   Slominski AT, Brożyna AA, Skobowiat C, et al. On the role of classical and novel forms of vitamin D in melanoma progression and management. J Steroid Biochem Mol Biol 2018; 177: 159-70.
[http://dx.doi.org/10.1016/j.jsbmb.2017.06.013] [PMID: 28676457]

[12]   Paolino G, Moliterni E, Corsetti P, et al. Vitamin D and melanoma: state of the art and possible therapeutic uses. G Ital Dermatol Venereol 2019; 154(1): 64-71.
[http://dx.doi.org/10.23736/S0392-0488.17.05801-1] [PMID: 29249122]

[13]   Wyatt C, Neale RE, Lucas RM. Skin cancer and vitamin D: an update. 2015; 2(1): 51–61. Available from: https://www.futuremedicine.com/doi/10.2217/mmt.14.31
[http://dx.doi.org/10.2217/mmt.14.31]

[14]   Raymond-Lezman JR, Riskin SI. Benefits and risks of sun exposure to maintain adequate vitamin D levels. Cureus 2023; 15(5): e38578.
[http://dx.doi.org/10.7759/cureus.38578] [PMID: 37284402]

[15]   Lu J, Sharma LK, Bai Y. Implications of mitochondrial DNA mutations and mitochondrial dysfunction in tumorigenesis. Cell Research. 2009; 19(7): 802–15.
[http://dx.doi.org/10.1038/cr.2009.69]

[16]   Jakupciak JP, Wang W, Markowitz ME, et al. Mitochondrial DNA as a cancer biomarker. J Mol Diagn 2005; 7(2): 258-67.
[http://dx.doi.org/10.1016/S1525-1578(10)60553-3] [PMID: 15858150]

[17]   Birch-Machin MA, Swalwell H. How mitochondria record the effects of UV exposure and oxidative stress using human skin as a model tissue. Mutagenesis 2010; 25(2): 101-7.
[http://dx.doi.org/10.1093/mutage/gep061] [PMID: 19955330]

[18]   Wartman D, Weinstock M. Are we overemphasizing sun avoidance in protection from melanoma? Cancer Epidemiol Biomarkers Prev 2008; 17(3): 469-70.
[http://dx.doi.org/10.1158/1055-9965.EPI-07-0301] [PMID: 18319330]

[19]   Nilsen LTN, Hannevik M, Veierød MB. Ultraviolet exposure from indoor tanning devices: a systematic review. Br J Dermatol 2016; 174(4): 730-40.

[http://dx.doi.org/10.1111/bjd.14388] [PMID: 26749382]

[20]   Lazovich D, Isaksson Vogel R, Weinstock MA, Nelson HH, Ahmed RL, Berwick M. Association Between Indoor Tanning and Melanoma in Younger Men and Women. JAMA Dermatol 2016; 152(3): 268-75.
[http://dx.doi.org/10.1001/jamadermatol.2015.2938] [PMID: 26818409]

[21]   Woo DK, Eide MJ. Tanning beds, skin cancer, and vitamin D: an examination of the scientific evidence and public health implications. Dermatol Ther 2010; 23(1): 61-71.
[http://dx.doi.org/10.1111/j.1529-8019.2009.01291.x] [PMID: 20136909]

[22]   Lopes FCPS, Sleiman MG, Sebastian K, Bogucka R, Jacobs EA, Adamson AS. UV exposure and the risk of cutaneous melanoma in skin of color. JAMA Dermatol 2021; 157(2): 213-9.
[http://dx.doi.org/10.1001/jamadermatol.2020.4616] [PMID: 33325988]

[23]   Fernández-García E. Skin protection against UV light by dietary antioxidants. Food Funct 2014; 5(9): 1994-2003.
[http://dx.doi.org/10.1039/C4FO00280F] [PMID: 24964816]

[24]   Dong Y, Wei J, Yang F, Qu Y, Huang J, Shi D. Nutrient-based approaches for melanoma: prevention and therapeutic insights. Nutrients. 2023; 15(20): 4483. Available from: https://www.mdpi.com/2072-6643/15/20/4483/htm

[25]   Brożyna AA, Hoffman RM, Slominski AT, *et al.* Relevance of vitamin D in melanoma development, progression and therapy. Anticancer Res 2020; 40(1): 473-89.
[http://dx.doi.org/10.21873/anticanres.13976] [PMID: 31892603]

[26]   Chlebowski RT, Johnson KC, Kooperberg C, *et al.* Calcium plus vitamin D supplementation and the risk of breast cancer. J Natl Cancer Inst 2008; 100(22): 1581-91.
[http://dx.doi.org/10.1093/jnci/djn360] [PMID: 19001601]

[27]   Stucci LS, D'Oronzo S, Tucci M, *et al.* Vitamin D in melanoma: Controversies and potential role in combination with immune check-point inhibitors. Cancer Treat Rev 2018; 69: 21-8.
[http://dx.doi.org/10.1016/j.ctrv.2018.05.016] [PMID: 29864718]

[28]   Zhang L, Wang S, Che X, Li X. Vitamin D and lung cancer risk: a comprehensive review and meta-analysis. Cell Physiol Biochem 2015; 36(1): 299-305.
[http://dx.doi.org/10.1159/000374072] [PMID: 25967968]

[29]   Baron JA, Barry EL, Mott LA, *et al.* A trial of calcium and vitamin D for the prevention of colorectal adenomas. N Engl J Med 2015; 373(16): 1519-30.
[http://dx.doi.org/10.1056/NEJMoa1500409] [PMID: 26465985]

[30]   Norman AW. From vitamin D to hormone D: fundamentals of the vitamin D endocrine system essential for good health. Am J Clin Nutr 2008; 88(2): 491S-9S.
[http://dx.doi.org/10.1093/ajcn/88.2.491S] [PMID: 18689389]

[31]   D'Oronzo S, Stucci S, Tucci M, Silvestris F. Cancer treatment-induced bone loss (CTIBL): Pathogenesis and clinical implications. Cancer Treat Rev 2015; 41(9): 798-808.
[http://dx.doi.org/10.1016/j.ctrv.2015.09.003] [PMID: 26410578]

[32]   Campbell MJ, Trump DL, Vitamin D. Vitamin D receptor signaling and cancer. Endocrinol Metab Clin North Am 2017; 46(4): 1009-38.
[http://dx.doi.org/10.1016/j.ecl.2017.07.007] [PMID: 29080633]

[33]   Yin L, Ordóñez-Mena JM, Chen T, Schöttker B, Arndt V, Brenner H. Circulating 25-hydroxyvitamin D serum concentration and total cancer incidence and mortality: A systematic review and meta-analysis. Prev Med 2013; 57(6): 753-64.
[http://dx.doi.org/10.1016/j.ypmed.2013.08.026] [PMID: 24036014]

[34]   Caini S, Gnagnarella P, Stanganelli I, *et al.* Vitamin d and the risk of non-melanoma skin cancer: A systematic literature review and meta-analysis on behalf of the italian melanoma intergroup. Cancers (Basel). 2021; 13(19).

[http://dx.doi.org/10.3390/cancers13194815]

[35]   Song Y, Lu H, Cheng Y. To identify the association between dietary vitamin D intake and serum levels and risk or prognostic factors for melanoma-systematic review and meta-analysis. BMJ Open 2022; 12(8): e052442.
[http://dx.doi.org/10.1136/bmjopen-2021-052442] [PMID: 36028262]

[36]   Balch CM, Soong ; Seng-Jaw, *et al.* An Evidence-based Staging System for Cutaneous Melanoma1. CA Cancer J Clin. 2004; 54(3): 131–49.
[http://dx.doi.org/110.3322/canjclin.54.3.131]

[37]   Balch CM, Gershenwald JE, Soong SJ. *et al.* Final version of 2009 AJCC melanoma staging and classification. Journal of Clinical Oncology. 2009; 27(36): 6199.

[38]   Wyatt C, Lucas RM, Hurst C, Kimlin MG, Vitamin D. Vitamin D deficiency at melanoma diagnosis is associated with higher Breslow thickness. PLoS One 2015; 10(5): e0126394.
[http://dx.doi.org/10.1371/journal.pone.0126394] [PMID: 25970336]

[39]   Borradale D, Isenring E, Hacker E, Kimlin MG. Exposure to solar ultraviolet radiation is associated with a decreased folate status in women of childbearing age. J Photochem Photobiol B 2014; 131: 90-5.
[http://dx.doi.org/10.1016/j.jphotobiol.2014.01.002] [PMID: 24509071]

CHAPTER 8

Vitamin D and Pregnancy

Shaikha Alnaqbi[1,*]**, Reem El Asmar**[1]**, Russul AlQutub**[1]**, Alyaa Masaad**[1]**, Noor Abu Dheir**[1]**, Salma Abu Qiyas**[1] **and Dimitrios Papandreou**[1]

[1] *Department of Clinical Nutrition and Dietetics, College of Health Sciences, University of Sharjah, Sharjah, UAE*

Abstract: Vitamin D insufficiency is prevalent among pregnant women and infants worldwide. Expectant mothers with a heightened risk of vitamin D deficiency may have notably low levels of 25-hydroxyvitamin D (25(OH)D) in their newborns, raising the likelihood of nutritional rickets. Numerous observational studies suggest a link between inadequate vitamin D levels during pregnancy and various adverse perinatal outcomes such as hypertensive disorders (like preeclampsia), restricted fetal growth, and premature birth. Nevertheless, the limited number of large-scale randomized controlled trials (RCTs) conducted so far have produced conflicting findings regarding the effectiveness of vitamin D supplementation in enhancing perinatal outcomes.

Keywords: Breastfeeding, Gestational diabetes, Pregnancy, Preterm, Preeclampsia, Supplement.

INTRODUCTION

Many nations have recognized vitamin D deficiency (VDD) as a public health issue; pregnant women are at a particularly high risk because their prevalence of VDD is up to 50% in the population [1]. Low vitamin D levels are common throughout pregnancy and infancy, however, there is limited information to establish dietary recommendations for vitamin D during these life stages [2]. Vitamin D is primarily responsible for preserving calcium homeostasis and promoting bone health. Furthermore, its involvement in various physiologic functions, such as immunomodulation, cell proliferation, and cell differentiation, has been established in numerous tissues and organs, including the heart, brain, and pancreas [3].

Recent research suggests that nutrition can influence immunological and metabolic programming during critical stages of fetal and postnatal development.

---

* **Corresponding author Shaikha Alnaqbi:** Department of Clinical Nutrition and Dietetics, College of Health Sciences, University of Sharjah, Sharjah, UAE; E-mails: U23102372@sharjah.ac.ae, shaikhaealnaqbi@gmail.com

Thus, modern dietary patterns may raise the risk of immunological and metabolic dysregulation, which is linked to an increase in a variety of noncommunicable diseases [4]. Vitamin D stands out among these nutrients; its impact on gene regulation and prenatal programming may describe its long list of health advantages [5].

Rickets in Newborns

Nutritional rickets remain a substantial global health concern among children, as evidenced by recent reports of its prevalence rising in numerous developed nations.

To avoid rickets, it is crucial for pregnant women and their infants to take vitamin D supplementation. Randomized controlled trials have shown that infants who receive 400 IU of vitamin D daily can reach 25-hydroxyvitamin D levels above 50 nmol/L [6].

Dental Consequences of Vitamin D

Research has shown that children whose mothers do not get enough vitamin D during the last three months of pregnancy are more likely to develop cavities in their permanent teeth by the age of six. On the other hand, there was no correlation between 25(OH)D in early life and the frequency or severity of enamel defects. In addition to bolstering the the established effects of vitamin D on bones and minerals, these findings add weight to the case for supplementation during pregnancy and the first few years of life [7].

VITAMIN D FOR MOTHER (PREECLAMPSIA, GESTATIONAL DIABETES)

There's a high prevalence of Gestational weight gain, gestational diabetes, and pregnancy-induced hypertension among women in developed countries [8, 9]. Vitamin D deficiency (VDD) poses a notable risk for pregnant women in Latin America, the Middle East, Asia, and Africa, with prevalence rates being the highest globally in these regions [10]. Maternal VDD is associated with an increased likelihood of various adverse health outcomes for both mothers and newborns. These include heightened risks of hypertension and gestational diabetes mellitus (GDM), elevated production of inflammatory cytokines of mother [11], insulin resistance, first cesarean section [12], high body mass index (BMI) of the mother as well as symptoms of postpartum depression [10].

A systematic review examined the links between maternal Vitamin D deficiency and pregnancy included six studies that utilized enzyme-linked immunosorbent assay (ELISA) methods [13 - 17], each revealing one or more positive associations between Vitamin D Deficiency (VDD) and maternal and/or neonatal health outcomes. Two of them demonstrated positive associations between VDD and maternal GDM [18], as well as neonatal low birth weight (LBW) and small for gestational age (SGA) [19]. Two studies focused on maternal outcomes and indicated a positive relation between VDD and maternal pre-eclampsia [20, 21], while the last two studies found no significant associations at all.

Vitamin D and Preeclampsia

Pre-eclampsia is a complex pregnancy disorder affecting multiple systems, characterized by varying levels of placental mal-perfusion that result in the release of soluble factors into the maternal circulation. These factors induce injury to the maternal vascular endothelium, giving rise to hypertension and multi-organ damage. The placental involvement in this condition can lead to fetal growth restriction and, in severe cases, stillbirth. Notably, pre-eclampsia stands as a significant contributor to both maternal and perinatal mortality and morbidity, particularly in low-income and middle-income countries [22].

In a cohort study involving 13,806 pregnant women, maternal vitamin D deficiency during the gestational period of 23 to 28 weeks was found to be strongly linked to an increased risk of severe preeclampsia. After adjusting for relevant confounding factors, the odds ratio (OR) was 3.16, with a 95% confidence interval (CI) ranging from 1.77 to 5.65 [21]. Notably, current research indicates that vitamin D supplementation has the potential to enhance nifedipine treatment for preeclampsia. This supplementation is shown to reduce the time required to control blood pressure and extend the duration before the occurrence of subsequent hypertensive crises, possibly through an immunomodulatory mechanism [23]. However, despite these positive effects, data on the preventive impact of vitamin D supplementation against the onset of preeclampsia in pregnancy remain inconclusive [24].

Vitamin D and Gestational Diabetes

GDM refers to the manifestation of diabetes symptoms during pregnancy in women who had normal glucose metabolism before becoming pregnant [25]. This condition is linked to an increased likelihood of developing type 2 diabetes mellitus (T2DM), metabolic syndrome (MS) and cardiovascular disease [26].

Women with GDM have a higher probability of undergoing cesarean deliveries, and their newborns tend to have a greater birth weight [27, 28] and a higher risk of childhood asthma [29]. GDM is also correlated with elevated risks of depression [30], childhood-impaired glucose tolerance [31], and childhood obesity [32]. Offspring born to mothers with GDM face an increased risk of developing T2DM during their teenage or early adult years [33]. The pathogenesis of GDM involves insulin resistance (IR) and reduced islet beta-cell secretion [34], and there is a notable association between GDM and low levels of vitamin D (VD) according to numerous studies [35].

In a recent meta-analysis encompassing data from 44 studies, which aimed to assess the connection between Vitamin D levels and the risk of gestational diabetes mellitus (GDM), findings were derived from a total of 37,838 pregnant women, including 6,694 diagnosed with GDM. The results indicated a notable association, suggesting that Vitamin D deficiency may contribute to the occurrence of GDM in pregnant women. Specifically, the 25-hydroxyvitamin D (25 (OH) D) levels in GDM patients were found to decrease by 5.14 nmol/L compared to the control group [36]. This outcome aligns with the results of previous meta-analyses on prospective studies, which consistently demonstrated a significantly reduced risk of GDM to higher levels of 25 (OH) D [37 - 39].

VITAMIN D FOR INFANTS

Given the prevalence of vitamin D deficiency among mothers, it poses a potential risk to the health outcomes of their offspring as well. Low birth weight (LBW), preterm birth (PTB), and being small for gestational age (SGA) are significant adverse birth outcomes, recognized globally as serious public health concerns [40, 41]. These outcomes contribute significantly to perinatal infant illness and death. Furthermore, infants born with LBW, PTB, or SGA face an increased risk of developing various chronic diseases later in life, such as diabetes and cardiovascular conditions [40]. Research indicates that multiple factors, including maternal nutrition, environmental influences, and genetic predispositions, can impact the occurrence of adverse birth outcomes, with maternal nutritional status during pregnancy being a potentially modifiable factor [42].

Numerous studies have examined maternal vitamin D status with the risk of PTB and SGA. A meta-analysis and systematic review of prospective studies reported an inverse association between maternal vitamin D status and the risk of LBW. A linear dose-response analysis revealed that for every increase in vitamin D serum level by 25 nmol/L, there was a corresponding decrease of 6% and 10% in the risk of PTB (respectively [43].

Another meta-analysis of 24 observational studies, encompassing cohort, case-control and cross-sectional studies, concluded that vitamin D deficiency during the first and last trimester may not have an effect on PTB, however, the important effect is more likely to happen during the second trimester PTB (OR = 1.33, 95%CI (1.15, 1.54), P = .000) [44]. Multiple studies have conducted clinical trials investigating the effect of vitamin D supplementation on the risk of PTB, LBW, and SGA. A systematic review evaluating randomized control trials and quasi-experimental studies published since 1995 concluded an improvement in the fetal outcome of PTB with the demonstration of vitamin D supplementation during pregnancy [45]. While another meta-analysis of randomized control trials reported no effect on the risk of PTB and LBW [46].

Vitamin D and Breastfeeding

Human milk is the ideal nourishment for babies. Breastfeeding is related to a lower incidence of viral and bacterial illnesses. Except for vitamin D, breast milk contains an ideal balance of nutrients for newborn growth. Vitamin D is essential for calcium metabolism and bone health, but it also has extra-skeletal effects, including innate immunity as well as adaptive immunity. Because exclusive breastfeeding possibly increases vitamin D deficiency, newborns should be supplemented with vitamin D during their first year of life. The awareness and adoption of breastmilk and vitamin D supplementation is an essential public health goal [47].

The suggested vitamin D dosage for nursing moms to improve their total vitamin D status, as a result, of their milk from breastfeeding, is (200-2,000 IU/day), reflecting a lack of consensus. Some research suggests that maternal high-dose supplementation with vitamin D (as much as 6,400 IU/day) might be utilised as an alternative to direct baby supplementation.

However, ongoing doubts exist over the effectiveness of high doses of Vitamin D supplementation for mothers. Direct baby supplementation is the only currently accessible approach for improving vitamin D levels in breastfed newborns. According to numerous associations and organisations around the world, the recommended daily amount of vitamin D for breastfeeding infants is (200-1,200 IU). Most worldwide guidelines indicate that newborns who are entirely or partially breastfed receive 400 IU of vitamin D per day for the first year of life.

To promote ideal infant development, growth, and health, the World Health Organisation (also known as the WHO) recommends exclusive breastfeeding for the first six months of life and introducing a safe and adequate nutrition at six months, and continued breastfeeding until two years of age or beyond [48].

Vitamin D Supplementation

Vitamin D supplementation during pregnancy has been a subject of ongoing debate for years. Issues of controversy surrounding supplementation with Vitamin D include optimal dosage regimens, safety considerations, the extent of benefits conferred, and the necessity of supplementation for all pregnant women *versus* solely those identified as deficient in vitamin D.

Initially issued in 2012, the WHO guidelines advised against Vitamin D supplementation during pregnancy for the prevention of pre-eclampsia and its associated complications [49]. WHO guidelines are updated periodically, as experts continue to examine emerging evidence from clinical trials on the administration of antenatal vitamin D supplementation. As of 2023, WHO maintains the position that vitamin D supplementation should not be recommended for all pregnant women for improvement of maternal and perinatal outcomes. However, the guidelines acknowledge that pregnant women suspected of vitamin D deficiency, including those residing in regions with limited sun exposure, may receive vitamin D supplementation at the current recommended nutrient intake (RNI) of 200 IU (5 µg)/d [50].

Recent reviews suggest that Vitamin D supplementation during pregnancy is needed in order to protect against adverse pregnancy outcomes. A review by Palacios and his colleagues found that supplementing pregnant women with vitamin D alone may decrease the risk of several adverse effects such as f pre-eclampsia, GDM, LBW, and severe postpartum haemorrhage [51]. Similarly, a recent review concluded that Vitamin D supplementation in pregnancy for vitamin D deficient women may enhance fetal growth and decrease the risk for gestational diabetes, preeclampsia, small-for-gestational-age, and preterm birth. The authors concluded that all pregnant women should receive a supplementation of 600 IU/day of vitamin D3. In addition, higher vitamin D doses (1000-4000 IU/day) may also be beneficial for better maternal and infant outcomes [52]. Several other recent reviews also highlighted the potential benefit of antenatal vitamin D supplementation on maternal and fetal outcomes [53 - 55].

With regard to safety, administering up to 4000 IU of vitamin D supplements during pregnancy appears to be generally safe. However, the criteria utilized to assess safety are sometimes unreported or vary across trials. It is imperative for future trials to maintain consistency in reporting adverse events to ensure comprehensive evaluation [54]

Generally, clinical trials investigating the efficacy of vitamin D supplementation during pregnancy have yielded promising results. That said, variations in the timing of supplementation, dosage levels, and methodological disparities across studies underscore the necessity for further research to determine the most effective supplementation strategy. Pregnant women are advised to consume balanced diets, like the Mediterranean diet, to ensure proper nutrition, as it has been proven to have positive effects and is widely regarded as the most effective method [50, 56].

CONCLUSION

Vitamin D defieciency has been shown to have adverse effects on pregnancy and infant health. Studies indicate that low levels of vitamin D during pregnancy can increase the risk of various complications such as hypertension, gestational diabetes, insulin resistance, heightened inflammatory responses and preeclampsia. Additionally, postpartum depression and higher maternal body mass index have been linked to vitamin D deficiency. Infants born to mothers deficient in vitamin D are more likely to be born prematurely, have low birth weight, or be small for gestational age. Therefore, it is essential to ensure adequate intake of vitamin D before conception through a well-balanced diet to mitigate these adverse effects, as supplementation during pregnancy has not been universally agreed upon to address these issues .Furthermore, introducing vitamin D supplementation or fortified foods to infants after six months of age becomes necessary, as breast milk alone does not meet the infant's vitamin D requirements beyond this age.

REFERENCES

[1]   Palacios C, Trak-Fellermeier MA, Martinez RX, *et al.* Regimens of vitamin D supplementation for women during pregnancy. Cochrane Libr 2019; 2019: (10).
[http://dx.doi.org/10.1002/14651858.CD013446] [PMID: 31581312]

[2]   Dutra LV. Souza FISd, Konstantyner T. Effects of vitamin D supplementation during pregnancy on newborns and infants: An integrative review. Rev Paul Pediatr 2021; 39.

[3]   Várbíró S, Takács I, Tűű L, *et al.* Effects of vitamin D on fertility, pregnancy and polycystic ovary syndrome—A review. Nutrients 2022; 14(8): 1649.
[http://dx.doi.org/10.3390/nu14081649] [PMID: 35458211]

[4]   Mansur JL, Oliveri B, Giacoia E, Fusaro D, Costanzo PR. Vitamin D: before, during and after pregnancy: effect on neonates and children. Nutrients 2022; 14(9): 1900.
[http://dx.doi.org/10.3390/nu14091900] [PMID: 35565867]

[5]   Pérez-López FR, Pilz S, Chedraui P. Vitamin D supplementation during pregnancy: an overview. Curr Opin Obstet Gynecol 2020; 32(5): 316-21.
[http://dx.doi.org/10.1097/GCO.0000000000000641] [PMID: 32487800]

[6]   Palacios C, Kostiuk LK, Peña-Rosas JP. Vitamin D supplementation for women during pregnancy. Cochrane Database of Systematic Reviews 2019; (7).

[7]   World Health Organization. Guideline: vitamin D supplementation in pregnant women. : World Health Organization; 2012.

[8]   Martin JA, Hamilton BE, Osterman MJ, Driscoll AK, Drake P. Births: final data for 2016. 2018.

[9]   Papandreou D, Mantzorou M, Tyrovolas S, *et al.* Pre-pregnancy excess weight association with maternal sociodemographic, anthropometric and lifestyle factors and maternal perinatal outcomes. 2022; 14(18): 3810.
[http://dx.doi.org/10.3390/nu14183810]

[10]   Shaw NJ. Prevention and treatment of nutritional rickets. J Steroid Biochem Mol Biol 2016; 164: 145-7.

[http://dx.doi.org/10.1016/j.jsbmb.2015.10.014] [PMID: 26493853]

[11]   Beckett DM, Broadbent JM, Loch C, Mahoney EK, Drummond BK, Wheeler BJ. Dental consequences of Vitamin D deficiency during pregnancy and early infancy—an observational study. Int J Environ Res Public Health 2022; 19(4): 1932.
[http://dx.doi.org/10.3390/ijerph19041932] [PMID: 35206117]

[12]   Vitamin D for health: a global perspective Mayo clinic proceedings. Elsevier 2013.

[13]   Prescott SL. Early nutrition as a major determinant of 'immune health': Implications for allergy, obesity and other noncommunicable diseases. Nestle Nutr Inst Workshop Ser 2016; 85: 1-17.
[http://dx.doi.org/10.1159/000439477] [PMID: 27088328]

[14]   Holick MF. Vitamin D deficiency. N Engl J Med 2007; 357(3): 266-81.
[http://dx.doi.org/10.1056/NEJMra070553] [PMID: 17634462]

[15]   McWhorter CA, Mead MJ, Rodgers MD, *et al.* Predicting comorbidities of pregnancy: A comparison between total and free 25(OH)D and their associations with parathyroid hormone. J Steroid Biochem Mol Biol 2023; 235: 106420.
[http://dx.doi.org/10.1016/j.jsbmb.2023.106420] [PMID: 37913892]

[16]   Mulligan ML, Felton SK, Riek AE, Bernal-Mizrachi C. Implications of vitamin D deficiency in pregnancy and lactation. Obstet Gynecol 2010;202(5):429. e1-429. e9.
[http://dx.doi.org/10.1016/j.ajog.2009.09.002]

[17]   Heo JS, Ahn YM, Kim ARE, Shin SM. Breastfeeding and vitamin D. Clinical and Experimental Pediatrics 2022; 65(9): 418-29.
[http://dx.doi.org/10.3345/cep.2021.00444] [PMID: 34902960]

[18]   Domenici R, Vierucci F. Exclusive breastfeeding and vitamin D supplementation: a positive synergistic effect on prevention of childhood infections? Int J Environ Res Public Health 2022; 19(5): 2973.
[http://dx.doi.org/10.3390/ijerph19052973] [PMID: 35270666]

[19]   Sadeghian M, Asadi M, Rahmani S, *et al.* Circulating vitamin D and the risk of gestational diabetes: a systematic review and dose-response meta-analysis. Endocrine 2020; 70(1): 36-47.
[http://dx.doi.org/10.1007/s12020-020-02360-y] [PMID: 32710437]

[20]   Poel YHM, Hummel P, Lips P, Stam F, van der Ploeg T, Simsek S. Vitamin D and gestational diabetes: A systematic review and meta-analysis. Eur J Intern Med 2012; 23(5): 465-9.
[http://dx.doi.org/10.1016/j.ejim.2012.01.007] [PMID: 22726378]

[21]   Milajerdi A, Abbasi F, Mousavi SM, Esmaillzadeh A. Maternal vitamin D status and risk of gestational diabetes mellitus: A systematic review and meta-analysis of prospective cohort studies. Clin Nutr 2021; 40(5): 2576-86.
[http://dx.doi.org/10.1016/j.clnu.2021.03.037] [PMID: 33933723]

[22]   Fatima K, Asif M, Nihal K, *et al.* Association between vitamin D levels in early pregnancy and gestational diabetes mellitus: A systematic review and meta-analysis. J Family Med Prim Care 2022; 11(9): 5569-80.
[http://dx.doi.org/10.4103/jfmpc.jfmpc_107_22] [PMID: 36505566]

[23]   Ede G, Keskin U, Cemal Yenen M, Samur G. Lower vitamin D levels during the second trimester are associated with developing gestational diabetes mellitus: an observational cross-sectional study. Gynecol Endocrinol 2019; 35(6): 525-8.
[http://dx.doi.org/10.1080/09513590.2018.1548593] [PMID: 30599810]

[24]   Liu Y, Hou W, Meng X, *et al.* Heterogeneity of insulin resistance and beta cell dysfunction in gestational diabetes mellitus: a prospective cohort study of perinatal outcomes. J Transl Med 2018; 16(1): 289.
[http://dx.doi.org/10.1186/s12967-018-1666-5] [PMID: 30355279]

[25]   Law KP, Zhang H. The pathogenesis and pathophysiology of gestational diabetes mellitus: Deductions

from a three-part longitudinal metabolomics study in China. Clin Chim Acta 2017; 468: 60-70.
[http://dx.doi.org/10.1016/j.cca.2017.02.008] [PMID: 28213010]

[26]   Purswani JM, Gala P, Dwarkanath P, Larkin HM, Kurpad A, Mehta S. The role of vitamin D in pre-eclampsia: a systematic review. BMC Pregnancy Childbirth 2017; 17(1): 231.
[http://dx.doi.org/10.1186/s12884-017-1408-3] [PMID: 28709403]

[27]   Pavlidou E, Papandreou D, Taha Z, *et al.* Association of maternal pre-pregnancy overweight and obesity with cAnthropometric factors and perinatal and postnatal outcomes: A cross-sectional study. 2023; 15(15): 3384.
[http://dx.doi.org/10.3390/nu15153384]

[28]   Lowe WL Jr, Scholtens DM, Kuang A, *et al.* Hyperglycemia and adverse pregnancy outcome follow-up study (HAPO FUS): maternal gestational diabetes mellitus and childhood glucose metabolism. Diabetes Care 2019; 42(3): 372-80.
[http://dx.doi.org/10.2337/dc18-1646] [PMID: 30655380]

[29]   Papandreou D, Pavlidou E, Tyrovolas S, *et al.* Relation of Maternal Pre-Pregnancy Factors and Childhood Asthma: A Cross-Sectional Survey in Pre-School Children Aged 2–5 Years Old. 2023; 59(1): 179.

[30]   Pace R, Rahme E, Da Costa D, Dasgupta K. Association between gestational diabetes mellitus and depression in parents: a retrospective cohort study. Clin Epidemiol 2018; 10: 1827-38.
[http://dx.doi.org/10.2147/CLEP.S184319] [PMID: 30584375]

[31]   Chiou YL, Hung CH, Liao HY. The impact of prepregnancy body mass index and gestational weight gain on perinatal outcomes for women with gestational diabetes mellitus. Worldviews Evid Based Nurs 2018; 15(4): 313-22.
[http://dx.doi.org/10.1111/wvn.12305] [PMID: 29962105]

[32]   Mantzorou M, Papandreou D, Pavlidou E, *et al.* Maternal gestational diabetes is associated with high risk of childhood overweight and obesity: a cross-sectional study in pre-school children aged 2–5 years. 2023; 59(3): 455.

[33]   Poola-Kella S, Steinman RA, Mesmar B, Malek R. Gestational diabetes mellitus: post-partum risk and follow up. Rev Recent Clin Trials 2018; 13(1): 5-14.
[PMID: 28901851]

[34]   Xu T, Dainelli L, Yu K, *et al.* The short-term health and economic burden of gestational diabetes mellitus in China: a modelling study. BMJ Open 2017; 7(12): e018893.
[http://dx.doi.org/10.1136/bmjopen-2017-018893] [PMID: 29203507]

[35]   Fogacci F, Banach M, Mikhailidis DP, *et al.* Safety of red yeast rice supplementation: A systematic review and meta-analysis of randomized controlled trials. Pharmacol Res 2019; 143: 1-16.
[http://dx.doi.org/10.1016/j.phrs.2019.02.028] [PMID: 30844537]

[36]   Chappell LC, Cluver CA, Kingdom J, Tong S. Pre-eclampsia. Lancet 2021; 398(10297): 341-54.
[http://dx.doi.org/10.1016/S0140-6736(20)32335-7] [PMID: 34051884]

[37]   Zhao X, Fang R, Yu R, Chen D, Zhao J, Xiao J. Maternal vitamin D status in the late second trimester and the risk of severe preeclampsia in southeastern China. Nutrients 2017; 9(2): 138.
[http://dx.doi.org/10.3390/nu9020138] [PMID: 28216561]

[38]   Hossain N, Kanani FH, Ramzan S, *et al.* Obstetric and neonatal outcomes of maternal vitamin D supplementation: results of an open-label, randomized controlled trial of antenatal vitamin D supplementation in Pakistani women. J Clin Endocrinol Metab 2014; 99(7): 2448-55.
[http://dx.doi.org/10.1210/jc.2013-3491] [PMID: 24646102]

[39]   Toko E, Sumba O, Daud I, *et al.* Maternal vitamin D status and adverse birth outcomes in children from rural Western Kenya. Nutrients 2016; 8(12): 794.
[http://dx.doi.org/10.3390/nu8120794] [PMID: 27941597]

[40]   Chen YH, Fu L, Hao JH, *et al.* Maternal vitamin D deficiency during pregnancy elevates the risks of

small for gestational age and low birth weight infants in Chinese population. J Clin Endocrinol Metab 2015; 100(5): 1912-9.
[http://dx.doi.org/10.1210/jc.2014-4407] [PMID: 25774884]

[41]   Maghbooli Z, Hossein-nezhad A, Karimi F, Shafaei AR, Larijani B. Correlation between vitamin D $_3$ deficiency and insulin resistance in pregnancy. Diabetes Metab Res Rev 2008; 24(1): 27-32.
[http://dx.doi.org/10.1002/dmrr.737] [PMID: 17607661]

[42]   Aydogmus S, Kelekci S, Aydogmus H, *et al.* High prevalence of vitamin D deficiency among pregnant women in a Turkish population and impact on perinatal outcomes. J Matern Fetal Neonatal Med 2015; 28(15): 1828-32.
[http://dx.doi.org/10.3109/14767058.2014.969235] [PMID: 25260128]

[43]   Gur EB, Gokduman A, Turan GA, *et al.* Mid-pregnancy vitamin D levels and postpartum depression. Eur J Obstet Gynecol Reprod Biol 2014; 179: 110-6.
[http://dx.doi.org/10.1016/j.ejogrb.2014.05.017] [PMID: 24965990]

[44]   Song SJ, Si S, Liu J, *et al.* Vitamin D status in Chinese pregnant women and their newborns in Beijing and their relationships to birth size. Public Health Nutr 2013; 16(4): 687-92.
[http://dx.doi.org/10.1017/S1368980012003084] [PMID: 23174124]

[45]   Ajmani SN, Paul M, Chauhan P, Ajmani AK, Yadav N. Prevalence of vitamin D deficiency in burka-clad pregnant women in a 450-bedded maternity hospital of Delhi. J Obstet Gynaecol India 2016; 66(S1) (Suppl. 1): 67-71.
[http://dx.doi.org/10.1007/s13224-015-0764-z] [PMID: 27651580]

[46]   Lapillonne A. Vitamin D deficiency during pregnancy may impair maternal and fetal outcomes. Med Hypotheses 2010; 74(1): 71-5.
[http://dx.doi.org/10.1016/j.mehy.2009.07.054] [PMID: 19692182]

[47]   Wei SQ, Qi HP, Luo ZC, Fraser WD. Maternal vitamin D status and adverse pregnancy outcomes: a systematic review and meta-analysis. J Matern Fetal Neonatal Med 2013; 26(9): 889-99.
[http://dx.doi.org/10.3109/14767058.2013.765849] [PMID: 23311886]

[48]   Van der Pligt P, Willcox J, Szymlek-Gay EA, Murray E, Worsley A, Daly RM. Associations of maternal vitamin D deficiency with pregnancy and neonatal complications in developing countries: a systematic review. Nutrients 2018; 10(5): 640.
[http://dx.doi.org/10.3390/nu10050640] [PMID: 29783717]

[49]   Gernand AD, Schulze KJ, Stewart CP, West KP Jr, Christian P. Micronutrient deficiencies in pregnancy worldwide: health effects and prevention. Nat Rev Endocrinol 2016; 12(5): 274-89.
[http://dx.doi.org/10.1038/nrendo.2016.37] [PMID: 27032981]

[50]   Global burden of prematurity. Seminars in fetal and neonatal medicine: Elsevier; 2016.

[51]   Liu L, Oza S, Hogan D, *et al.* Global, regional, and national causes of child mortality in 2000–13, with projections to inform post-2015 priorities: an updated systematic analysis. Lancet 2015; 385(9966): 430-40.
[http://dx.doi.org/10.1016/S0140-6736(14)61698-6] [PMID: 25280870]

[52]   Liu Y, Ding C, Xu R, *et al.* Effects of vitamin D supplementation during pregnancy on offspring health at birth: A meta-analysis of randomized controlled trails. Clin Nutr 2022; 41(7): 1532-40.
[http://dx.doi.org/10.1016/j.clnu.2022.05.011] [PMID: 35667269]

[53]   Oh C, Keats E, Bhutta Z. Vitamin and mineral supplementation during pregnancy on maternal, birth, child health and development outcomes in low-and middle-income countries: a systematic review and meta-analysis. Nutrients 2020; 12(2): 491.
[http://dx.doi.org/10.3390/nu12020491] [PMID: 32075071]

[54]   Zhao R, Zhou L, Wang S, Yin H, Yang X, Hao L. Effect of maternal vitamin D status on risk of adverse birth outcomes: a systematic review and dose–response meta-analysis of observational studies. Eur J Nutr 2022; 61(6): 2881-907.

[http://dx.doi.org/10.1007/s00394-022-02866-3] [PMID: 35316377]

[55] Lian RH, Qi PA, Yuan T, *et al.* Systematic review and meta-analysis of vitamin D deficiency in different pregnancy on preterm birth. Medicine (Baltimore) 2021; 100(24): e26303.
[http://dx.doi.org/10.1097/MD.0000000000026303] [PMID: 34128867]

[56] Antasouras G, Papadopoulou SK, Alexatou O, *et al.* Adherence to the mediterranean diet during pregnancy: Associations with sociodemographic and anthropometric parameters, perinatal outcomes, and breastfeeding practices. Medicina (Kaunas) 2023; 59(9): 1547.
[http://dx.doi.org/10.3390/medicina59091547] [PMID: 37763666]

SUBJECT INDEX

A

Absorption 33, 40, 61, 84
  intestinal 40
  postprandial glucose 33
Acute respiratory distress syndrome (ARDS) 26
Adaptive immunity 16, 18, 22, 104, 113
Adipocytes 40, 47
Adipokines 35, 40
  inflammatory 40
Adolescents, obese 38
Adrenal medullary cells 6
Age 2, 7, 19, 23, 34, 39, 44, 103, 105, 110, 111, 112, 113, 115
  gestational 111, 112, 115
  -related effect 103
Aging processes 92, 99
Air-polluted areas 2
Airway(s) 24, 25
  chronic 24
  obstruction 25
Akkermansia 72
Albuminuria 50
Alveolar 25
  abnormalities 25
  epithelium 25
Amino acids, essential 18
Analogs 4, 5, 23
  natural 4
  synthetic 5
Anti-apoptotic properties 44
Anti-cancer effects 6
Anti-fibrotic effect 25
Anti-inflammatory 41, 49, 64
  effect 64
  processes 49
  properties 41
Anti-microbial peptides 22
Anti-proliferative actions 101
Anti-rachitic 3, 4
  activity 4

factor 3
  properties 3
Antidepressants 85, 91
Antimicrobial 17, 18, 19, 22, 25, 72
  activity 22
  effects 25
  peptides 17, 18, 19, 72
Antirachitic factor 3
Anxiolytic effects 85
Asthma control 24
Atherosclerosis 44, 60, 61, 63, 64, 65, 67
Athletes 7, 62
  older 62
  young 62
Autoimmune 16, 18, 19, 20, 21, 22, 23, 24, 26, 101
  conditions 18, 21
  diseases 16, 19, 20, 21, 22, 23, 24
  disorders 16, 18, 20, 26, 101
Autophagy down-regulation 40

B

Balance, neurotransmitter 86
Basal cell carcinoma (BCC) 103
Beck depression inventory (BDI) 89
Behavior problems 88
Behavioral modifications 100
Bipolar disorder 88
Bladder cancer 97
Blood 46, 65, 66, 88, 91, 99, 102, 103, 104
  maternal 88
Blood pressure (BP) 6, 44, 50, 61, 65, 66
  diastolic 50
  homeostasis 61
  lower 66
  systolic 65, 66
Body 19, 39, 40, 41, 43, 47, 105, 110
  fat 40
  mass index (BMI) 19, 39, 40, 41, 43, 47, 105, 110
Bone 2, 5

www.ingramcontent.com/pod-product-compliance
Lightning Source LLC
Chambersburg PA
CBHW041446210326
41599CB00004B/144